LifeDetox ☺

First published in Great Britain in 2007 by
Piatkus Books Ltd
5 Windmill Street, London W1T 2JA
email: info@piatkus.co.uk

A catalogue record for this book is available from the British Library

ISBN 978 0 7499 2796 7

Text design by Smith & Gilmour Ltd London

This book has been printed on paper manufactured
with respect for the environment using wood from
managed sustainable resources

Printed and bound in Italy by EuroGrafica SpA, Marano Vicenza

Contents

To both of our mums, dads and bros,
and the beautiful gift that is Jana.

Acknowledgements

Thanks to my parents who have unfailingly supported my life path, with all its twists and turns. To friends and family scattered throughout the world that have loved and taught me so much, and with special thanks to François, a great friend and yoga teacher, for his fantastic photos for this book. For detox clients who never cease to bring great pleasure and inspiration. To the experience of Vipassana for the peace and insights that make sense of it all. To Jana, whose smile says it all. And to Sandy, a loving reminder to enjoy the joy.
Amanda

Thanks to my parents for their love and support, along with my teachers and friends scattered throughout the world for sharing their wisdom and honesty. Thanks also to my coaching and therapy clients, workshop and retreat attendees – you have all taught and inspired me so much. Special thanks to Amanda and daughter Jana – you are both amazing.
Sandy

We would also like to thank Gill Bailey and Jo Brooks of Piatkus for all their brilliant advice and support, and our copy editor Jan Cutler for her excellent work in editing.
Sandy and Amanda

☺

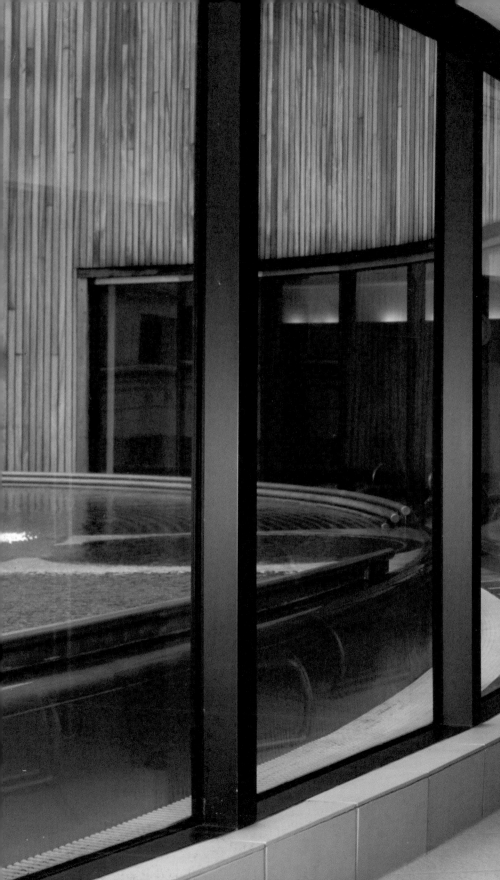

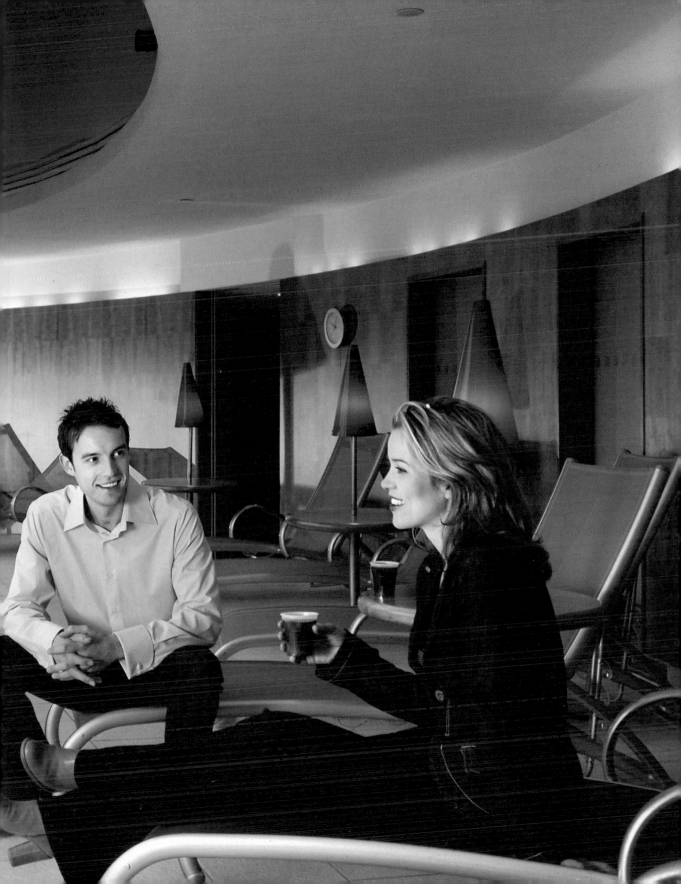

Welcome to Life Detox

Before we explain about the 7-day detox programme, which is the core of our Life Detox, here is a little about how each of us learned about detox and how we discovered together that detoxing the mind as well as the body can have an amazing effect.

Amanda's story

While I was in my teens and early twenties, I was a classic case of someone who although not ill did not feel that great either. I was young with the world at my feet but I had symptoms that were undermining my energy, self-esteem and vitality.

For many years I suffered with bad skin and had tried several courses of antibiotics that helped, but when the tablets were finished so the problem returned. Knowing that it was the drugs that were making my skin look better made me feel like a fraud. It was around this time that I started reading about the toxic side-effects of antibiotics and was outraged to discover that the irritable bowel syndrome (IBS) symptoms that I had suffered with could be a side-effect of taking the medication.

Since I was 16 I had represented Scotland at badminton, and needed to maintain a suitable weight for my sporting career. However, I would crave carbohydrate foods such as bread and cereals, making this hard. I tried eating low-calorie foods, processed cereals with skimmed milk and drinking diet drinks – but I later learned that this combination was a nightmare for my body.

The cycle continued throughout my early twenties when I began to work in television. As you can imagine, there is a considerable pressure to look good on TV, and, yes, it is true, the camera does add 10 pounds to your weight! It wasn't until I began to study nutritional medicine that things took a dramatic turn. What I was reading changed my outlook forever. I ditched the diets and gave up listening to what commercials and clever marketing told me would keep me slim. Instead, I began eating real food, not processed foods or diet foods, and a remarkable thing happened: my symptoms started to clear up almost immediately. I studied furiously, trying out detox techniques and nutrition plans that supported my liver (the main fat-burning organ of the body) and my digestive system so that my body could effectively 'clear out'. My skin looked better than it had done in years; my bloating left – and my self-confidence returned. And most amazing of all, I lost weight without trying!

I qualified as a nutritionist in my early twenties, and over the years in clinical practice began to see that the vast majority of people needed more than just a diet plan – they needed a detox. I would become frustrated at the lack of progress in some cases until I came to the realisation that you are not what you *eat* but you are what you *absorb*. You may take lots of expensive supplements, probiotic drinks, and use other lotions and potions, but unless your body is working well, you may as well pour your money down the drain. The toxic load that the average body carries around is so great that it can impair any effort to lose weight, improve a health condition or simply gain more energy.

'You are not what you eat but you are what you absorb.'

Eventually I quit the clinic and travelled to Spain to set up a healing detox retreat – it was to be an inspired decision. I was able to develop a greater understanding of people's needs and learned that no matter how effective the physical detox was, without an emotional counterpart the process was incomplete. The final piece of the jigsaw fell into place when I met Sandy. He was able to explain how the mind–body connection worked, and, more importantly, he put together therapies and programmes to help people detox emotionally as well as physically. The results were incredible! Our holistic approach took our work to a whole new level.

Now held in numerous countries, our detox retreats have developed and improved over time. It has been rewarding to see people from all walks of life arrive at the retreat on day one in need of a detox, and then to see them leave on day seven looking and feeling ten years younger. But I am aware that there are only so many people that can come to the retreat; what about the millions of people who need help now? That is where *Life Detox* comes in. This book is the culmination of my journey, both personal and professional. I hope you enjoy the freedom and wisdom that *Life Detox* brings as much as I do.

Amanda

Amanda Hamilton

Sandy's story

As a child I was absolutely terrified of reading out loud in class. So much so that I would dread going to school, and I had a very negative association with reading in general. It wasn't until age 15 that I finally read a book from cover to cover. As it happens, it was a self-help book! From then on I was hooked. Through my mid- to late teens I devoured personal development and mind, body and spirit books, and I quickly became known as the guy who would have something useful to say if you had a problem. What's more, I got a real buzz whenever people confided in me.

However, despite my 'self-help toolkit' overflowing with some really useful stuff, I failed to get round to applying any of it to my own life. This led to a pretty turbulent time – both mentally and emotionally – as I struggled my way up the hill of my early twenties. Then, I could best be described as lonely, insecure and bored (not to mention inwardly irritated at most things). Don't get me wrong, life wasn't that bad; it was OK, but that was the point: it was *just* OK.

Feeling uncomfortable in my own skin with the uneasy feeling that *'There must be more to life than this!'*, I did the obvious thing: I trained and then began practising as a life coach!

I noticed a trend in the type of clients I was attracting: they all wanted my help to feel different – whether it was more calm, confident or content, purposeful, passionate or positive. This inspired me to train in Neuro Linguistic Programming (NLP), Time Line Therapy® and Meridian Therapy, and to specialise in helping people to clear their 'emotional baggage' and take charge of their emotional destiny.

During this time I decided to sort out my own skeletons. I worked with a coach to bring to the surface and clear my emotional hurts and improve my confidence. To my delight I immediately started to attract amazing opportunities into my life. Speaking of which, I met Amanda. We immediately clicked both personally and professionally.

My approach has always been to work with my clients to help them get to the root cause of their problems, instead of dealing solely with the surface-level symptoms. This approach complemented Amanda's body detox work beautifully. By combining the body detox with techniques to clear negative thoughts and emotions, we found our clients benefited from genuine and long-lasting changes.

In 2006 I featured alongside Amanda on UKTV's most successful home-grown series to date, *Spa of Embarrassing Illnesses*, in which we helped eight people to cure their conditions by detoxing their body and mind at our stunning Turkish detox retreat. Today, Amanda and I work together throughout Europe giving talks, writing and running the Life Detox retreats.

As you work through the fantastic body detox outlined in this book, I urge you to include the mind detox too. You will learn about the constant interplay between your mind and your body and I will share a number of practical ways to help you feel more consistently calm, confident and content. Quite literally, you can change your mind to get the body and life you want. I use these techniques with my clients at my clinic in the UK and retreat centres around the world with amazing results.

You bought this book for an important reason (or perhaps a number of reasons), so please don't just read it and say, 'That's nice, I really should do that one day.' I encourage you to make the commitment to yourself to get what you want, not only from this book but also from your body and your life – starting today!

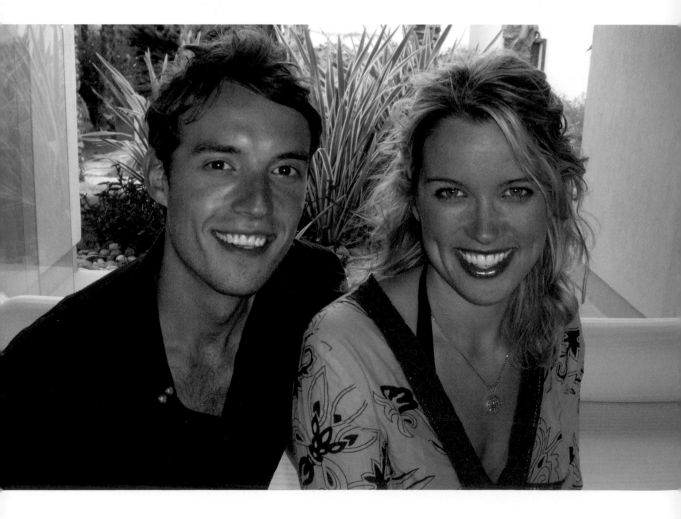

Sandy Newbigging

Our story: Life Detox

Our hands on training at retreats, workshops and clinics, combined with our studies of nutritional medicine and the power of the mind, have given us the depth of experience to create an easy to follow and effective Life Detox programme for you. Our numerous happy and healthy clients are testimony that it works.

Detox is the ultimate feel-good tool for the 21st century. Our aim is to make our detox easy and accessible for you, whether you are busy with career demands or deep in the rough and tumble of family life. Use *Life Detox* to navigate your way through a major turning point in your life. With its cutting-edge detox principles you can enter into a world where perfect health, mental clarity and feeling great can become your way of life. And the best part of it all is that anyone can do it!

We have successfully helped every type of person – from overweight to underweight, from sick to those reaching for ultimate health and performance. Our programme has changed lives and made lives – where couples needed some help with their fertility, our detox principles have led to many healthy little detox babies. This Life Detox programme is our passion: a simple answer to so many needs. It has changed the way we live our lives forever. Here are just some of the ways it has helped others, too:

☺ Permanent weight loss.
☺ Dramatic improvements from chronic health conditions.
☺ Enhanced energy levels and an overall feeling of vitality.
☺ Clearer skin, including the improvement of conditions such as acne, psoriasis and eczema.
☺ Sharpened senses and mental clarity.
☺ Reduced blood pressure and improved cholesterol levels.
☺ Improved fertility in both men and women.
☺ Cleaner living and working environments.
☺ Enhanced confidence in self and others.
☺ Freedom from the past and optimism about the future.
☺ Massively reduced stress and anxiety levels.

Our incredible Life Detox 7-Day Programme has the power to transform your body, your mind and your life. It achieves this by not only helping you to clear physical toxins, but also mental and emotional ones.

'I embarked on the detox hoping to jump-start a healthier lifestyle. What I achieved was a whole new life. I feel fantastic – calmer but with more energy and a healthy, happy glow. I have stopped smoking without using patches, lozenges or gum. And if that wasn't enough, the mind detox also cut me loose from feelings of guilt and fear that had plagued me for more than a decade. It's amazing that something so simple can be so successful.' Lindsay Clydesdale, women's editor for the *Daily Record*

Each day of your Life Detox moves you towards a healthier and happier body and mind. You will find that many other, seemingly unrelated, aspects of your life improve, too. Life Detox gets such fantastic results because it takes account of the fact that you are much more than just a physical body. Your body, mind and lifestyle are all connected and have an impact on each other. We have found that no cleanse is complete unless you detox them all. A body-focused detox programme may help you shift a few pounds, but what happens the next time you get stressed or when unresolved emotional issues resurface? You reach for the biscuit tin or a glass of wine, right? If you want to let go of mental or emotional blocks once and for all, then this book can change the way you think and feel forever.

By applying what's outlined in the following pages you will know, perhaps for the first time, how it feels to have a mind and body that help you to create the life you want.

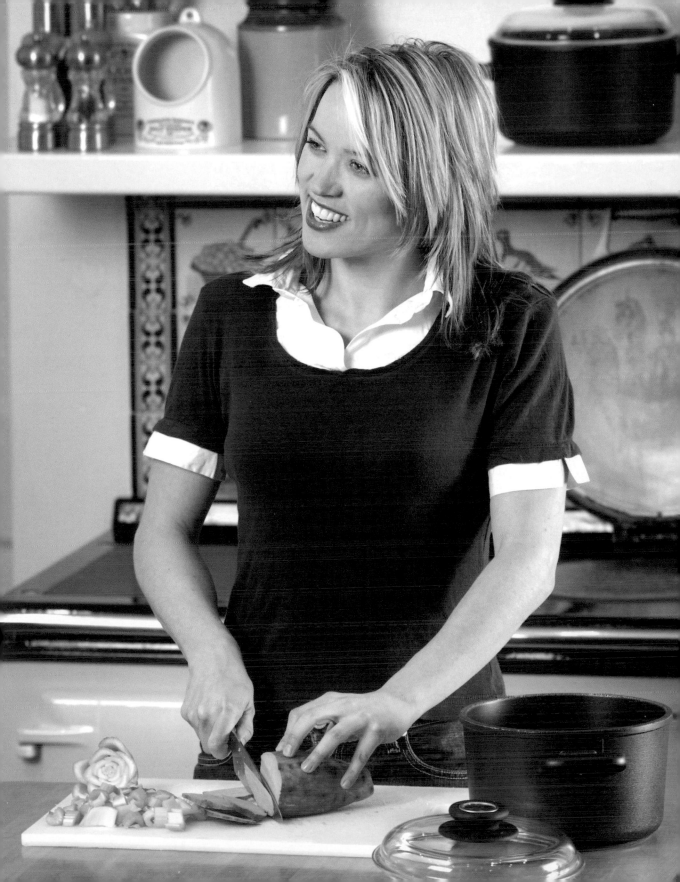

How to use this book

Although you will be keen to start, please don't be tempted to turn straight to the Life Detox 7-Day Programme.

Background and planning

Part 1 tells you all you need to know about the toxic lifestyle that most of us lead today and how we can benefit from cutting down our exposure to toxins, as well as reducing stress and toxic emotions in our lives.

At the beginning of Part 2 we explain how to prepare for your Life Detox 7-Day Programme, including the best time to start, your shopping list and optional ideas to turbocharge your detox.

The 7-Day programme

Chapters 9 and 10 introduce you to our exercise options, the Life Detox themes and the daily programme. This is followed by the detox itself.

Each day of the detox has its own schedule, which lists the exercises we have planned for you as well as the food you will be eating. The ingredients for each day's juice or smoothie are listed in the details that follow the schedule; the recipes for our suggested meals, however, can be found at the end of Part 2 on pages 123–141.

The detox is intended to fit around a normal working day. We've designed it to be as stress-free and enjoyable as possible.

Continuing with the new you

Part 3 concentrates on your new healthy life and begins with an optional concentrated turbo-detox day of juice fasting. This day is not intended to fit around a workday. If the idea of an extended detox appeals to you, please read Chapter 12 before you embark on the programme. The remainder of Part 3 looks at maintaining maximum health by keeping your mind free of stress and emotional toxins.

We hope you will enjoy your Life Detox, and that it will be the beginning of a new way of living for you.

partone [1]
why you need
a life detox

We Are All Toxic

In our modern world we are exposed to environmental conditions and chemicals that are detrimental to our health. Combine that with negative thinking or our inability to cope with difficult past experiences or concerns about our future and we have a body that is susceptible to discomfort and illness. All these negative influences are toxins, which put our health and well-being under threat.

Your body under threat

Whether you believe it or not, you are incredible. From your largest organs to your smallest cells, every part of your body interacts with each other. Your system regulates itself subtly every second of every day, according to what you eat, drink, breathe, think, feel or do. As you are reading this sentence, 50,000 of the cells in your body will die and be replaced with new cells. Your liver, which is your main organ of detoxification, has over 500 different specialist functions, and scientists are still discovering more. Nerve impulses that help you to move your hand when you turn the page, or reach out for your cup of tea, travel to and from the brain as fast as 340 miles per second. In fact, your body is designed to protect you from any kind of danger, internal or external. But, it doesn't always work so beautifully.

Trying to keep up with environmental changes

Our bodies have evolved over millions of years to cope with a whole host of threats; yet, our recent history has changed the landscape of our lives completely. Billions of kilos of man-made chemicals make their way into the eco-system of the planet 24 hours a day, which means that the average man and woman are absorbing a multitude of chemicals every day. Until 150 years ago, these chemicals did not exist, but now they are found in food, drugs (both social and medical), water, air, cosmetics, the soil, household goods, gardens and public recreation areas such as parks and swimming pools.

If you are like the majority of people we see in our clinics or on our detox retreats, your body could be struggling with a range of basic functions such as digestion, immunity and weight control that can be traced back to a lifestyle that is continually putting your body under toxic stress. Your skin, too, is a reflection of your internal health, so if is not glowing and peachy then it's time to take action.

The majority of people will fall into one of the following two categories:

Type 1

You eat according to healthy guidelines most of the time, you go to the gym or take regular exercise. Basically, you do most things 'right' according to what you have read and watched on television, and yet you still don't look or feel amazing. It could be an irritating problem that just won't go away: perhaps a few pounds that just won't shift, or skin that suffers from outbreaks of spots or rashes every now and then. It could be any niggling issue – it does not mean that you are ill but that you have not yet reached your full, healthy potential.

Type 2

You are suffering from a 21st-century condition that, no matter what medication you have taken or advice you have followed, just won't go away. By 21st-century condition we mean that the symptom or symptoms you are experiencing are lifestyle related.

Here's a shortlist of the most common: IBS or other digestive complaints; weight gain; candida (thrush); fungal infections; cystitis; headaches; mood swings; fatigue; allergies; hormone imbalances; infertility or recurring miscarriages; chronic fatigue; high blood pressure; Type II diabetes or hypoglycaemia (low blood sugar); skin problems; high cholesterol; emotional eating; stress; addictions (to sugar, caffeine, nicotine, alcohol); insomnia; painful joints.

What do each one of these conditions and complaints have in common? The answer is that they are all related to the level of toxins that have built up in your body. Symptoms will vary according to each individual's genetic predisposition and how much they have been exposed to toxins, but the source of the problem is the same. Understanding a little of how your body works, what toxins are and how your body can become toxic will give you a good grounding when you come to do the Life Detox 7-Day Programme, so read on.

What is a toxin?

A toxin is anything that has a detrimental effect on cell function or structure – in other words, it prevents the body from working well. These toxins come from a variety of sources, yet the common factor between all of them is that they are man-made synthetic chemicals which are foreign to our bodies.

It's important to distinguish these man-made chemicals from toxins created by the human body. The body itself can produce toxins; they are a natural by-product of its day-to-day functioning. When the body is overloaded with toxins it is unable to get rid of them effectively and a build-up appears, often with the onset of an irritating health problem that just won't go away. Antibiotics and a poor diet, for example, can upset the internal gut bacteria balance, which can then become toxic over time causing symptoms such as yeast infections.

Our lifestyle

The vast majority of toxins that build up in our bodies come from our lifestyle, with processed foods being the biggest culprit. Processed foods contain artificial additives, preservatives and stabilisers, artificial colouring and flavouring, harmful trans-fats and high levels of added sugar and salt. The average person's daily diet can also expose them to industrial chemicals such as pesticides and herbicides, alcohol, environmental hormones and toxic heavy metals.

The unborn child is also affected by environmental assaults, and it is of such concern that, in the UK, the Food Standards Agency (FSA) recommends that pregnant women limit or even avoid tuna and swordfish, often thought of as healthy foods, due to the worrying levels of toxins from mercury, polychlorinated biphenyls (PCBs) and dioxins, which can negatively effect the developing foetus. We recommend eating any fish only in moderation (no more than twice a week). Although known for its healthy omega-3 oils, the dangers of toxins in fish have led many nutritionists to conclude that vegetable proteins should make up a larger part of most people's diets.

Another toxic assault on our bodies comes from drugs. Although it is well known that drugs (including nicotine and caffeine) are toxic, not everyone is aware that over-the-counter medication or prescriptions from your doctor are also sources of toxins in themselves.

The invisible overload

Once your body's own detoxification system becomes overloaded, toxins that have accumulated over a period of time can wreak havoc on normal metabolic processes such as weight control and the immune system. Most toxins do not have a dramatic, immediate and noticeable effect, and therefore their effects remain untreated. Toxins accumulate and damage the body in hidden ways, day in and day out, and the level to which your body is burdened by them is called your toxic load.

Your toxic load

The toxic load describes the level of toxins you have accumulated in your life up until now. For example, if you are currently a smoker or heavy drinker then your 'load' is likely to be greater than somebody who does not smoke and has only the occasional glass of wine. But there are many hidden ways that people become toxic (see Chapter 5: Take Our Toxic Tests), so even if you have practised a fairly healthy lifestyle, the chances are that you have a toxic load which would be best dumped. Until your system gets the MOT and service that a detox provides, then your body's systems for keeping you in tip-top shape cannot do their job properly.

Today's overloaded body

Have you ever stopped to think carefully about what you eat, drink or breathe in one day? At the current time it is estimated that 2,000 new industrial chemical substances make their way into our bodies each year, through the food we eat, the water we drink and the air we breathe – and the number is growing, fast. And that is on top of the estimated 80,000 chemicals in our lives already. To put this into perspective, just two generations ago the chances are that in your family household there were virtually no processed foods in the cupboard, all household cleaning was done with natural substances, and 'air freshener' meant opening the windows – and, of course, there were no mobile phones. Common house dust contains a mixture of pesticides, heavy metals, flame retardants, solvents and hormone-disrupting chemicals. They form an invisible toxic hazard that scientists have only just begun to study, but we have been inhaling them since the day we were born.[1]

Here are some of the less well-known environmental threats to your health:

Plastics in food packaging, water bottles, and so on, contain harmful chemicals that can leach into your food. Even the toys children play with can put their health at risk.[2]

Non-stick coating on pans and other kitchenware is suspected to be toxic as it can emit fumes, which have been known to kill pet birds and make people sick.[3] Aluminium pans can also leach toxins into the food.

Pesticides and other gardening products contain chemicals, which you absorb through your skin and lungs.

Electrical equipment omits potentially cancer-causing electromagnetic fields (EMFs). Ill health has also been widely reported from people who live beneath overhead power cables.

Mobile phones contain chemicals that have a melting temperature close to 37°C (98.6°F), the temperature of the human body. Body heat and moisture from your body can increase the amount of chemicals released when the phone is used, which can enter the body through the lungs or skin. Symptoms include tiredness, headaches, blushing and dizziness, as well as allergies and cancer.[4] It is also suspected that men who spend more than four hours a day on a mobile phone have significantly lower sperm counts due to the electromagnetic radiation from the phones.[5]

On the more positive side, though, your body has the capability of changing from moment to moment and you can shed your toxic load; all you need is the knowledge to do so.

Detox and lose weight

Your body has to get rid of fattening chemicals if you want the chance to have the body you desire in the long term. This requires the help of the liver and the colon, the two organs essential in the battle of the bulge.

1 Support your liver
The main organ of detoxification and breaking down fat in the body is the liver. What this means is that a toxic or overloaded liver (sometimes called a 'sluggish' liver) can actually cause weight gain. However, the liver is not able to work effectively if it lacks certain nutrients from the food you eat or if it is

congested with man-made chemicals. Eating a poor diet means that not only are you not getting enough of the vitamins, minerals and essential fats that your body needs to work well, but also that the toxins in the food you eat can drain your body of essential nutrients – a toxic vicious cycle.

Many so-called diet products or foods are so toxic to the liver that they can hinder the very breakdown of fat they are sold to address. Signs of a toxic liver linked to weight gain include cellulite, weight gain around the abdominal area, gallstones and bloating. During the Life Detox there is a strong emphasis on supporting the liver with nutrients and specialist combinations of foods.

2 Clear your digestive system

Don't believe the popular saying, 'You are what you eat'. The truth is that you are what you *absorb*. What this means is that you have to be able to gain access to the goodness in the food you are eating for your body to be 'fed' properly. If you have any kind of digestive complaint, then most likely your body is not absorbing the goodness as it should. If your body is not getting enough nutrients it will send the signal for you to eat more – a classic way in which people gain weight. This problem is made all the worse if you regularly eat processed foods, which are difficult for your body to digest and lacking in nutrients.

What happens next is that unless you are able to eliminate waste effectively, it builds up into what is called 'colon plaque'. This can weigh several pounds! It is not pleasant and can lead to serious health problems such as 'leaky gut syndrome', in which the toxic waste that is stuck in your body gradually penetrates the gut wall, allowing foreign substances into the blood stream. Digestive complaints are the most common conditions that are treated in our detox clinic – and the biggest shock is that the majority of people don't even realise they have them.

Healthy moves

If your system is working optimally, each part of the body will receive what it needs with minimal toxic residue left behind. Did you know that unless you have between one and three well-formed bowel movements daily you are constipated? The journey of your food from one end to another is called 'transit time' and this process takes between 24 and 48 hours in a healthy person. Yet from our experience with clients, the average person has a transit time of approximately 65 to 100 hours!

If you want to get an idea of your body's average transit time, eat a portion of fresh beetroot (either cooked, grated raw or juiced) and then wait. The beetroot will stain your faeces and the time between consumption and elimination will tell you the approximate transit time.

Additional support

There is no point in struggling with diets until you detox and help your body to work better from the inside out. The Life Detox 7-Day Programme will support your nutritional needs, but if you have had a weight problem for a long time we suggest you use the detox supplements (see page 68) at the same time for additional support. Also make sure you follow the long-term guidelines for your mind and body.

Hidden allergies and 21st-century diseases

Just one generation ago allergies and intolerances were unusual. Two generations ago they were practically unheard of. These days allergies and intolerances are commonplace. Symptoms of a classic allergy are dramatic, and the chances are that if you have an allergy you already know about it. The dangerous peanut allergy is a good example of this. However, the much more common phenomenon of food intolerances can cause a great deal of stress and symptoms in the long term, and are usually not so immediately obvious. Common foods that cause intolerances are dairy produce, wheat, caffeine (found in tea, coffee, chocolate and cola drinks), red wine and yeast. Many people are allergic or intolerant to wheat, and suffer from symptoms such as bloating and gas. These symptoms clear up effortlessly when the offending items are removed from the daily diet.

During a detox you need to give your body a break from these stresses, so if you suspect you have an allergy or intolerance it is well worth finding out what is triggering your symptoms. Typical symptoms of allergies and intolerances include asthma, gastro-intestinal symptoms (nausea, vomiting, bloating and diarrhoea), eczema, urticaria (hives), sneezing and a runny nose. Other more long-term symptoms can include depression, anxiety, fatigue, migraine, sleeplessness and hyperactivity in children.

Testing for an allergy or food intolerance

There are two tests: the Classical Allergy test, or MAST IgE test, which is used for immediate allergic responses (such as the sudden and violent reaction to nuts); and the FoodScan IgG test, used for food intolerance. The food intolerance test involves taking a tiny sample of blood and is quick and easy to do in your own home (see Suppliers and Further Resources), whereas the allergy test needs to be done under the supervision of a healthcare professional.

What next?

Once you have isolated the problem food you can remove it from your diet. The next step to take is to improve your digestion, something that the Life Detox 7-Day Programme will really help you with.

Your mind can be toxic, too

Although your mind, like your body, is incredible, it can, nevertheless, become toxic.

The average person has as many as 90,000 thoughts every day. Some of these thoughts pass through your mind with little or no impact upon your body or life. The rest fall into two categories: thoughts that help you and thoughts that hinder you. The ratio between these positive and negative (toxic) thoughts depends largely upon the conclusions you've come to during your life. These are conclusions you've made about who you are and what you can and cannot be, do and have, and also conclusions about other people and the world you live in.

Do you get stressed easily? Do you have low self-confidence? Do you feel that you just have to look at a bar of chocolate to wear it on your hips? These are all examples of toxic conclusions that can prevent you creating and enjoying the body and life you want.

Freely flowing emotions

Emotions can become toxic, too. Emotions are in effect 'energy in **motion**' within your body. They are designed to flow around your body without obstruction. However, it is possible for them to become stuck in your system. Negative emotions – such as anger, sadness, fear, guilt, hurt and grief – are the most common emotions to become stuck, because most people resist feeling them. These stuck emotions are energy that has become stagnant in your system. If emotions remain stagnant, over time they may become toxic. By clearing them you can reduce the toxic load on your mind and body.

chapter two

Mr and Mrs Toxic

Meet Mr and Mrs Toxic. The chances are you will be able to relate to elements of their toxic lifestyle, because they represent a large proportion of the population today. Their bodies bulge with excess fat. They have harmful habits, such as smoking, and both feel stressed from the demands of work and family life. They are surrounded by toxic cleaning and cosmetic products and they fuel themselves with large amounts of processed food and fizzy drinks.

Smoking
Apart from damaging the lungs, smoking affects the digestive system,[7] liver, kidneys and immune system, and it reduces the skin's ability to regenerate, slowing the rate at which wounds heal and increasing the rate of ageing.

Bad breath and body odour
Both bad breath and poor body odour are signs of a toxic body.

Stress
Mental and emotional stress have been found to cause biochemical changes in the body, elevate stress hormone levels, speed up the ageing process and even reduce the effectiveness of the immune system.

Beer belly
Processed foods and alcohol are full of empty calories and toxins, putting your body under a double dose of stress. Overeating and binge drinking help fuel the growth of the beer belly, a body shape that puts men at increased risk of heart disease and diabetes.

Bloating and constipation
These are signs of a toxic bowel. A detox helps your system to clear out and can improve digestion.

Falling sperm count
Sperm counts among men have fallen by 29 per cent over the past 12 years,[6] a drop that has been blamed on obesity, smoking, stress, pollution and 'gender-bending' chemicals, which disrupt the hormone system.

MR TOXIC

In the home
Mr and Mrs Toxic also use a variety of cleaning products for their home and pesticides to maintain the garden. By using natural alternatives their exposure to toxins would be dramatically reduced (see Suppliers and Further Resources).

Poor sleeping patterns
The mind uses those times when you are mellow and quiet, such as when you are asleep, to try to resolve emotional problems. This can disrupt your sleep. Poor sleeping patterns can, therefore, be a symptom of a toxic mind.

Skin problems
Acne and hives are a sign of an overloaded liver and a need to detox.

Cellulite
Known as 'toxic fat', cellulite affects around 95 per cent of women. Detox helps to clean the body from the inside, helping to improve the appearance of skin.

Beauty products
The average woman buys some kind of beauty product each week – whether it is skin care, hair care, make-up or perfume. These are usually loaded with chemicals. (See Suppliers and Further Resources for natural alternatives.)

Falling fertility
One in every four pregnancies miscarries. A nutritional detoxification and preconception programme has been shown to improve fertility and the likelihood of successful pregnancy. In two groups of women who were having difficulty conceiving, one group followed a detox programme and 55 per cent had successful pregnancies; the other group underwent IVF and only 22 per cent had successful pregnancies.[8]

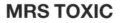

MRS TOXIC

chapter three

How Life Detox Works

Life Detox cleanses both the mind and body to strengthen the immune system and provide a feeling of health, vitality and well-being.

Give your body a break

Detoxification itself is actually a natural body process, not something that needs to be medically induced. Your body forces you to rest and eat lightly when fighting a virus or infection – it gives your system the chance to use more of its energy for dealing with the problem rather than coping with the demands of heavy digestion or stress. For example, when your nose is streaming from a cold or you are 'sweating out' a fever, this is your body detoxing naturally. When the body is healthy it is able to keep the balance right – the toxic input and output are the same. However, with exposure to a particular toxin or a gradual build-up of toxins, problems can occur. If your toxic load is light you will probably have little or no side-effects, but that does not mean it is not worth detoxing. By undertaking a detox *before* illness takes hold, you are taking a proactive approach – your body is your vehicle and it will work much better with some investment in its fine tuning.

A detox needs internal energy

Are you familiar with the 'Christmas dinner' or heavy meal? The caricature of a family slumped lethargically in front of the television, half asleep, illustrates perfectly the way the body copes with a big meal. By sending you to sleep it gets more energy to cope with the monumental task of breaking down the food and drink consumed. If you eat a light meal instead, the internal energy that is left over can be used to dispose of unwanted toxins in the body.

The Life Detox 7-Day Programme couples a light and easy-to-digest diet with nutrient-rich foods (with the option of supplements) to support your body's natural cleansing process. Toxic substances such as caffeine, alcohol and additives are removed to give your liver time to rejuvenate.

The detox boosters (see page 58) are designed to support your body's elimination – of toxins further. The main organs of elimination – the gastrointestinal tract (or digestion), the liver, the kidneys, the blood, lymphatic system, the lungs and the skin – are all given specific tools to support their function. These tools vary from a sauna, to help your skin eliminate toxins more effectively, to breathing techniques that will enhance the oxygenation of the tissues in the body.

Why the detox diet works

Hippocrates (c.460–377BC), the founding father of modern medicine, famously stated: 'Let food be thy medicine'. Health and vitality can be achieved through understanding which foods work best for your body. It's not about calorie counting, it is about getting the body in balance from the inside out.

Nature's science: acid–alkaline balance

pH is a measure of the acidity or alkalinity of a substance. It is measured on a scale of 0 to 14. The lower the pH the more acidic the substance; the higher the pH the more alkaline the substance. Keeping the body's blood and tissues in an alkaline state is beneficial for health.

The effects of unbalanced pH
The Western diet is acid-forming and so the majority of people who suffer from an unbalanced pH are too acidic. The following foods can put your body into a more acidic state:

☹ Processed foods
☹ Too many dairy products

- ☹ Caffeine
- ☹ Alcohol
- ☹ Smoking
- ☹ Salt
- ☹ Too much meat
- ☹ Carbonated drinks
- ☹ Sugar (either added to food or in processed foods)

An acidic body requires extra minerals to buffer (neutralise) the acid and safely remove it from the body. But because these minerals are deficient in the average diet they are often taken from stores held in vital organs and the bones. The strain of pH imbalance takes its toll on the body and plays a part in the development of 21st-century diseases such as those listed below:

- ☹ Cardiovascular problems
- ☹ Weight gain, obesity and diabetes
- ☹ Bladder and kidney conditions, including kidney stones
- ☹ Low immunity
- ☹ Hormone disruption
- ☹ Premature ageing
- ☹ Osteoporosis
- ☹ Joint pain, aching muscles and lactic acid build-up
- ☹ Low energy and chronic fatigue
- ☹ Slow digestion and elimination
- ☹ Yeast/fungal overgrowth

Life Detox selects foods that are not only alkaline-forming but are also rich in life-giving vitamins and minerals. Our recipes provide real food with real flavour, so the need for sugar, salt or processed additives is dramatically reduced.

The mind–body connection

Cleaning the body is vital, but until unhelpful habits, behaviours or toxic emotions are also cleansed, the process can be incomplete. And for that you need to deal with the realm of the mind. What do the following all have in common: crying when upset; laughing when amused; and getting a red face when embarrassed? They are all everyday examples that prove your mind and body have a direct and immediate impact on each other. In recent years, scientists have been able to prove that your thoughts and feelings affect your body. When you speak to yourself, the trillions of cells that make up your body hear *and* respond accordingly. Your body has an influence on your mind and, equally, your mind affects your body, and it does so seamlessly and subtly every moment of every day. Life Detox works because it takes into account that your mind, body and lifestyle all influence each other.

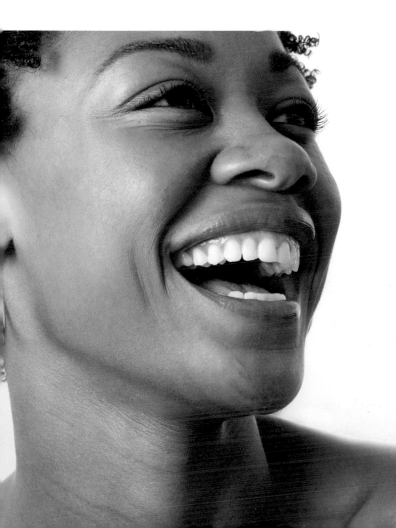

casestudyAlex ☺

When we met Alex he worked as a Royal Marine. His body was the example of the perfect male specimen. He could run for miles, ate only the best foods and looked after his body extremely well. However, he had an embarrassing illness that was ruining his life. He suffered from hyperhydrosis, a condition that meant he sweated profusely, drenching the clothes he wore and the sheets he slept upon. He always had to take a change of clothes everywhere he went and even had to sleep on a towel. Despite being successful at anything he turned his hand to, the condition was making him feel like a failure. It had an impact on all areas of his life. His time out with his friends was constantly overshadowed by his condition. He was even planning to leave his job because he was up for promotion but felt he couldn't attend the formal events due to his excessive sweating.

He had tried everything, including an operation, which had only made the condition worse. Then he attended a Life Detox retreat with us. During our time together he became aware that, for many years, he had been carrying around a massive amount of anxiety about what people thought of him. He would worry all the time and feel nervous anytime the spotlight was on him. Through mind exercises and body boosters (see page 76) we helped him to stop worrying about what other people thought of him. As a result he became more comfortable in his own skin. On day five of the Life Detox retreat, after suffering from hyperhydrosis for many years, he finally stopped sweating heavily – and to this date, has successfully been able to control it.

Alex is not an isolated case. We have repeatedly found through our work at our clinics and international retreats that people's physical conditions often improve when they deal with their unresolved emotional issues. These blocked emotions can become toxic and play a role in creating dis-ease within the person's body, and illustrate that if you want to change your body or your life, cleansing your mind is as important as any physical clear-out.

The power of your mind

How else might your mind be able to affect your body? Many scientists have investigated this exact question. One study found that after just five minutes of 'caring and compassionate' thoughts, the levels of volunteers' immune systems had risen significantly, taking five hours to return to the levels they were before the experiment.[9] Futhermore, the same study found that thoughts of 'anger and frustration' reduced the levels of the volunteers' immune systems for the same period. But the impact of your mind doesn't stop there.

The body responds to the mind

Your mind has the power to influence the size, shape, look, feel and overall health of your body and life. When you think and feel positive, your body responds by creating positive physical conditions. However, the opposite also happens when you think and feel negatively. It is for this reason that taking account of your mental and emotional well-being is vital when making changes to any physical conditions.

Your conscious and unconscious mind

Tune into your mind for a moment by noticing your thoughts. The ones you can hear have made their way up to your conscious awareness. They exist in what's called your conscious mind. However, there is also a part of your mind that operates below the surface of conscious awareness, and you are unconscious of this during your day-to-day life. Your unconscious mind performs many remarkable tasks without you having to be aware of them. It runs and heals your body, helps you make sense of life events, stores your memories, generates your emotions and drives your behaviour. Knowing how your unconscious mind works is the equivalent of getting your hands on the user manual for your body and life. You become able to clear your 'emotional baggage', improve your mental alertness, live without stress and anxiety more easily, and much more.

Life Detox works with the mind–body connection, combined with an understanding of how your mind works. During the Life Detox 7-Day Programme you will complete a series of proven exercises and detox boosters to help you to change your body and life by changing your mind.

Here are some key principles about Life Detox:

Life Detox is *not* like a traditional diet

As most people who have been on diets are acutely aware, diets don't work. How many people do you know who have lost and then regained weight on a calorie-controlled diet? Most fad diets restrict the intake of essential nutrients and essential fatty acids (EFAs) from foods such as nuts and seeds, which are needed to help your body work efficiently, including fat metabolism itself.

Life Detox works in a different way: *with* your body and mind rather than against them. When your body begins to work more effectively it can cleanse the existing toxins and deal with future toxins more efficiently. When your mind develops more clarity and you become more self-aware, any bad habits that have been undermining your emotional and physical well-being can be let go of once and for all.

What you will find

Your Life Detox 7-Day Programme is easy to follow and includes tasty juices, smoothies and recipes, body and mind exercises, and detox boosters. You wake up each day with a juice or smoothie and energise yourself throughout the day with raw power snacks, a liver-loving lunch and a detox dinner. Finally, you have the option to seal in the results by using a couple of detox boosters in the evening. It's specially designed to give your body and mind time to relax and re-energise, even while holding down a full-time job or other commitments. You are going to love how it makes you look and feel.

chapter four

Detox's Amazing Benefits

Look around you. How many people do you know who feel energetic, happy and full of vitality, and who glow with health? Our guess is that they are few and far between. The fact is that 99 per cent of us could feel a lot better than we do right now.

When I, Amanda, first began to work as a nutritionist it was not my intention to spend my time detoxing people all around the world. But, as the first clinic grew in popularity, so did my resolve to get to the root cause of people's conditions. In fact, it soon became apparent that unless you detox the mind as well as the body, the effects of a change of diet are often simply dealing with the surface of a problem.

If we told you what to eat but did not attempt to deal with the underlying emotional cause of your eating behaviour, would we be helping you to solve the real problem? No. If we changed your diet in an attempt to help you lose weight, despite the fact that your colon was full of impacted toxic waste and your liver was struggling under its toxic load, would we be helping solve the real problem? No. The Life Detox 7-Day Programme can help you benefit from the following:

1 Weight loss and reduction in cellulite

Losing excess weight is a welcome side-effect of the detox for most people. The initial shift in weight can be quite significant and will become steadier if you carry on with the programme long-term, according to how much weight there is left to lose.

Cellulite is also known as 'toxic fat', a sign of a congested inner environment, and it gathers mainly around the hips, thighs and bottom areas. This dimpled fat can be reduced when the fat cells (where toxins are often stored) are reduced. If you suffer from cellulite, make sure you do the optional skin-brushing detox booster (see page 58), as this can bring an immediate improvement in the texture of the skin. Also try to include as many of the detox superfoods into your Life Detox as possible (see page 65).

Your body shape is controlled by your hormones, and toxins interfere with the functioning of these hormones. Besides the obvious change in size with weight loss, a change of body shape is a welcome side-effect of reducing the toxins in your body. For men, most change is seen around their middle, whereas women will notice a reduction in excess fat from the waist, hips and thighs.

casestudySharon☺

Sharon is a very busy mum of three with a full-time job. When we first met her she was tired, overweight, with cellulite, and was feeling depressed. Within two months of the detox and follow-on maintenance diet she lost 12.7kg (2 stone/28lb).

'I have never felt physically better. I followed the detox programme and the follow-on diet almost to the letter and it has changed how my whole family eats – as well as changing my outlook on life! I feel more able to be a good mum, as well as being good to myself.' *Sharon, 30*

casestudyColin☺

Colin was approaching 40 and had developed a taste for junk food since his divorce four years ago. The resulting large, unsightly beer belly put him at increased risk of heart disease and diabetes. He was depressed and wanted his younger and fitter self back.
'I will admit that when we first started the diet I was a bit sceptical – I've seen all the diets promising untold changes and amazing weight loss but yours

definitely worked. I was astounded at not only the weight loss of 1½ stone [9.5kg] but also the energy that returned to me. I used to be fit when I was younger but I never dreamed it would still be achievable at nearly 40. Friends who hadn't seen me for a while were dumbstruck at the difference. Oh, and my mum really, really thanks you, as she was convinced I was heading for a heart attack!' *Colin, 39*

2 Reduced blood pressure and cholesterol

Amanda has had amazing results with changes in blood pressure and cholesterol on this detox programme, and has even astounded doctors. By reducing saturated fats and sodium – both associated with processed foods – and increasing the intake of fibrous fruit and vegetables as well as essential fatty acids, the body has the nutrition it needs to put itself back into balance. If you have either of these conditions, also try to include the detox supplements (see page 68) in your diet, as these can really help. However, medication should not be altered without the guidance of your health-care practitioner.

'I have seen how Amanda's diet produces transformational health benefits which are as powerful as the strongest drugs; for example in reducing cholesterol. But just as important is the effect on well-being. Her approach adds years to life and life to years.' Professor Ian Philp, MD and Government Tsar on Ageing

3 Improved skin

The skin is an organ of elimination, and a chronic skin condition is a signal of inner problems. If the problem is acne then the reduction in hormone residues from toxic food will certainly help, alongside using organic products for your skincare and organic foods for your diet in general. Conditions such as eczema or psoriasis often have genetic predispositions, but even so, it is possible to alleviate and even remove symptoms of skin problems through detoxification. If you have been on steroid medication for such a condition then it is even more important that you follow the liver support advice given on page 69. As the mind and body impact each other, stress can also have a big impact on the skin.

'I was a complete self-diagnosed "stress head" ... until I did a Life Detox retreat. I can confidently say that I am a much more relaxed person now and a number of the negative health side-effects of the stress have completely disappeared – accompanied by the drastically improved appearance of my skin. I feel brilliant!' Melissa Porter, TV presenter

4 Enhanced vitality

We could all do with more energy at times, but it is when we become tired of being tired that we need to worry. Imagine how it would feel to have energy all of the time, no matter what is happening in your life. Vitality is a gift you give yourself if you invest just a bit of that energy into detoxing every now and again.

5 Improved digestion

Because it's what you absorb that is important, money spent on nutritional supplements can be wasted if your own internal drainage system is so clogged up that certain nutrients cannot be absorbed. Toxins can leak from a sluggish gut directly into the bloodstream, causing allergy-type symptoms, lethargy and headaches. Your bowel habits might not make such good dinner conversation, but improving your bowel function could make a huge difference to every aspect of your health.

6 Improved fertility for women and men

It is estimated that one in seven couples have problems conceiving or maintaining a healthy pregnancy. Nutrition is fundamental to preparing the body for successful conception and is vital for the developing baby. We have had a lot of success with 'detox babies', as they have come to be known, and have quite a little photo gallery of cute baby pictures.

Detox is a natural, easy and cheap way to help boost your body's ability to conceive and carry a baby successfully to full term, but both partners need to do this to achieve the benefits. In short, a healthier mum and dad will make a healthier baby. In a comparative study provided by Foresight (the society for the promotion of preconception health), an improved diet coupled with detoxing to remove residual toxins produced the following amazing results:

☺ Seventy-eight per cent of couples who were having difficulty conceiving had healthy babies after detoxing, compared to 22 per cent of couples from another group who used IVF.
☺ Only 3.5 per cent of 'detox pregnancies' end in miscarriage, compared to 25 per cent of the NHS national average.
☺ Of the 'detox babies', 0.47 per cent were born with malformations compared to 6 per cent of the NHS national average.

Note You should detox before getting pregnant, not during pregnancy. Ideally, begin a detox programme three months before trying for a baby.

Detox is not only important if you have had fertility issues in the past. If you want to give your baby the healthiest start, a detox is helpful. Amanda conceived after a detox programme and, although she was not aware of any fertility problems, it helped her to rest assured that her system had been cleared of residual toxins that could affect a developing baby.

casestudyCaroline ☺

'I had been experiencing a variety of health problems for many years, despite the fact that I was only 29. IBS and period problems were the main issues, although my skin was also prone to teenage-style "break-outs". However, it was after having a miscarriage and spending a year trying to get pregnant again that I finally felt motivated to contact Amanda …She put me on a detox (which my partner also followed) and told me to identify any unresolved issues such as lingering infections or hidden allergies. I started to feel better almost immediately and wanted to try for a baby straight away, although Amanda was keen that I keep to a follow-on programme for a few more weeks to iron out some health issues. When we started trying again I fell pregnant straight away! I experienced none of the sickness of my first pregnancy and am delighted to say I had a happy, healthy and gorgeous little boy nine months later.'
Caroline, 29

7 Relief from chronic health problems

However your health problem has been labelled, whether migraine, IBS or stress, it is classed as a chronic problem. This means that you will have been experiencing the symptoms for a while, possibly years. Whereas most of the time people believe they will just have to learn to live with their problem, why not solve the issue once and for all? Detox works at the root cause of problems, solving issues from the inside out.

8 Heightened immune system

Like all systems in your body, your immune system gets a boost when it is fed the right nutrients. The Life Detox diet is jam-packed with vitamins and antioxidants essential for keeping your immune system working well.

Also, try following our recommendations for incorporating more caring and compassionate thoughts into your daily life, as this has also been found to have a positive impact on immune-system levels.

9 Mind benefits

If you're carrying around a truckload of toxic thoughts about who you are, what you can't be, or what you can't do or have, you will severely limit your enjoyment in life and your success. Also, if you're holding on to a lifetime of unresolved negative emotions, you can experience dis-ease within both your body and your mind. By detoxing your mind when detoxing your body you can:

☺ Free yourself from toxic emotions, such as anger, sadness, fear, guilt and grief.
☺ Stop bad habits and change conclusions that corrode your life enjoyment and success.
☺ Reduce stress and feel calm, confident and content in any situation.
☺ Resolve conflict with your family, friends and colleagues.
☺ Enhance mental clarity and creativity for massively improved results.

Life Detox is the ultimate tool for 21st-century living. Welcome to your detox journey.

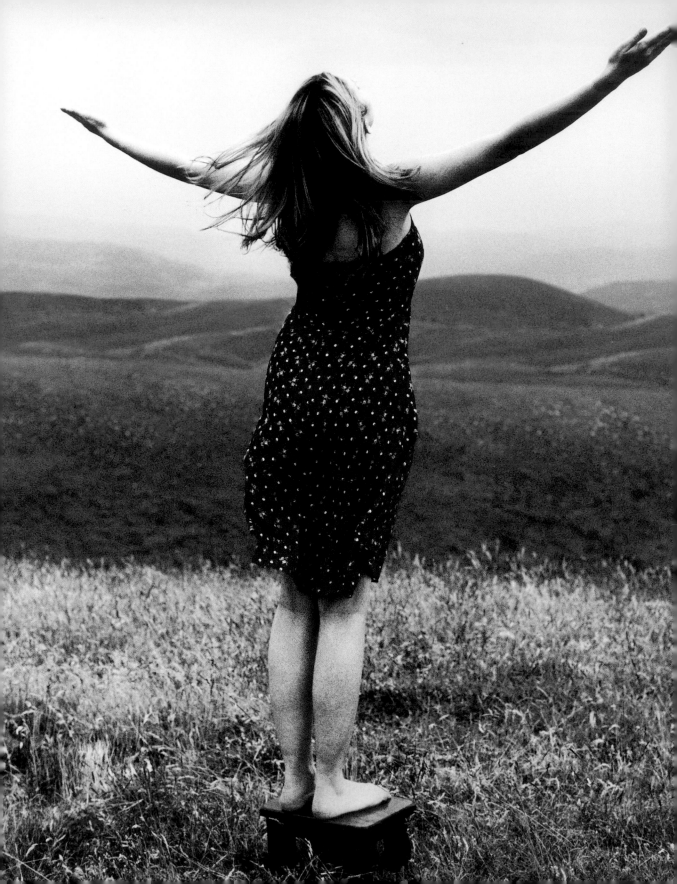

chapter five

Take Our Toxic Tests

Because of our modern lifestyle, it is unlikely that your body has been untouched by toxins. You may be surprised to learn that some of the foods you eat and everyday items you use can add to a build-up of toxins which affect your health and well-being. Take our tests to see how at risk your body is. If you answer yes to any of them, you would benefit from a detox.

Toxic body test

Diet

These foods contain elements that can either cause intolerances or allergies, or build up in our bodies producing all kinds of minor ailments that stop us from feeling full of vitality. Do you eat/drink any of the following on a regular basis:

① Processed food such as ready meals, bread, canned food, biscuits, crisps, cakes, chocolate or sweets? ☐
② Non-organic meat and/or fish? ☐
③ Salt or salty substances (including soy sauce) added to meals? ☐
④ Sugar or sweeteners added to drinks or food? ☐
⑤ Non-organic dairy produce – milk, cheese, butter, cream, ice cream? ☐
⑥ Unfiltered tap water? ☐
⑦ Drinks that contain caffeine? ☐
⑧ Decaffeinated drinks? ☐
⑨ Carbonated drinks? ☐
⑩ Alcohol? ☐
⑪ Juice for diluting or cordials that contain additives? ☐

Symptoms of a Toxic Body

Related to a toxic liver

☹ Cellulite

☹ Nausea after eating fatty foods

☹ Weight gain around the abdomen or excess weight

☹ Mood changes/foggy brain/depression

☹ Allergies such as hives, rashes, asthma

☹ Headaches

☹ High blood pressure

☹ Menstrual disturbances/early onset of the menopause

☹ Hypoglycaemia/low blood sugar

☹ Gallstones

☹ Chronic fatigue syndrome

☹ Excessive body heat

☹ Bad hangovers

☹ Hormonal imbalances

☹ Infertility

☹ Breast pain

Related to toxic digestion

☹ Whitish or yellowish mucus on the tongue (mostly mornings)

☹ IBS symptoms

☹ Constipation

☹ Bloating

☹ Loose stools most of the time

☹ Acid reflux

☹ Belching/passing wind frequently

☹ Difficult bowel movements

☹ Faeces like 'rabbit droppings'

If you are suffering from any of the conditions listed on the chart above then *Life Detox* has come at a good time – your body needs to reduce its toxic load.

Cooking and storage

We are exposed to chemicals and carcinogens simply by the methods we choose to cook or store our foods. If you use any of the methods below you will have absorbed toxins that a detox can help to remove.

① Do you store food in plastic containers or cling film? ☐
② Do you use a microwave? ☐
③ Do you barbecue food more than once a month? ☐
④ Do you frequently cook at high temperatures, such as roasting? ☐

Other ways toxins can reach us
Are you aware that the following represent toxic threats to your body? How many apply to you?
1. Do you have any mercury fillings in your teeth?
2. Have you had cosmetic surgery or enhancement, including botox?
3. Do you regularly use cosmetics and perfume?
4. Do you smoke cigarettes or cigars?
5. Do you take drugs of any kind, including medical drugs or the pill?
6. Do you use a mobile phone?

At home and in the workplace

Turning now to your home, garden and working environment, there are many chemicals and other toxins that you might be in contact with. Look at the following list:

① Do you clean with bleach, disinfectant and detergent? ☐
② Do you have MDF, chipboard, fibreboard or plywood in your home? ☐
③ Do you have stain-resistant or fire-retardant finishes on your curtains or furniture? ☐
④ Have you recently painted any rooms in your home or is your paintwork more than 20 years old? ☐

⑤ Do you use pesticides in your garden? ☐
⑥ Do you live in the countryside where fields are sprayed with pesticides? ☐
⑦ Do you live near power cables from pylons or a mobile phone mast? ☐
⑧ Do you live near to a flight path? ☐
⑨ Do you live in a city? ☐
⑩ Do you work in an air-conditioned office? ☐
⑪ Do you work with chemicals of any kind? ☐
⑫ Do you work with electrical equipment such as photocopiers for long periods of time? ☐

Toxic mind test

Your mind can become toxic due to internal feelings as well as external factors such as your relationships, how you react with others and how you manage your life at work and at home. Look at the lists below to see if any of the points apply to you.

Internal feelings

① Do you often find it hard to make decisions? ☐
② Do you have difficulty concentrating? ☐
③ Do you often feel irritable or snap at others? ☐
④ Do you consider yourself to be a fearful person who worries excessively? ☐
⑤ Do you find it hard to express your feelings? ☐
⑥ Do you put yourself down and/or allow others to? ☐
⑦ Do you feel dissatisfied with your life to the point of envying others? ☐
⑧ Do you find it hard to be still and relax? ☐
⑨ Do you have trouble sleeping, wake frequently, or suffer from nightmares? ☐

⑩ Do you still feel tired when you wake in the morning? ☐

⑪ Do you often want to cry and/or find it hard to cry? ☐

⑫ Do you feel guilty about things you should, or should not, have done? ☐

Other factors

① Do you have family conflict? ☐

② Do you watch more than one hour of television each day? ☐

③ Do you avoid visiting the dentist and/or doctor? ☐

④ Do you often miss deadlines and/or turn up late for appointments? ☐

⑤ Do you take things for granted? ☐

⑥ Do you have unpaid bills, taxes, debts or fines? ☐

⑦ Do you have difficulty communicating? ☐

⑧ Do you have bad habits that you want to change? ☐

⑨ Do you avoid taking exercise? ☐

⑩ Do you feel you are on 'information overload'? ☐

⑪ Do you drink more alcohol than you think is healthy? ☐

You will probably have found several points in the lists above that apply to you. If so, you definitely need to reduce your toxic load. Now read on to discover how you can do this.

chapter six

15 Top Detox Tips to Get You Started

1 Avoid eating wheat. This means cutting out biscuits, bread, cakes and pasta, and checking the labels on the food you buy, because wheat is found in many processed foods. Even if you are not intolerant to wheat, it remains one of the most difficult foods to digest. Instead, eat oatcakes, rice cakes, rye bread, wheat-free bread, rice, quinoa, buckwheat and spelt.

2 Avoid dairy – that is, milk, cheese, ice cream and cream. Don't worry about your calcium intake; you get more calcium from green vegetables! Small amounts of butter and eggs are fine. Instead of cow's milk drink soya milk, rice milk, quinoa milk, oat milk or almond milk and eat soya yogurts. Goat's products, such as feta cheese, can still be used sparingly.

One of the ways in which animals remove toxins is through their milk which is why dairy products contain toxins. The average cow is given chemicals designed to make it gain weight faster. The toxic cocktail includes steroids and antibiotics as well as pesticide residues.

3 Choose organic food where possible. Organic produce is free from pesticides and harmful additives. It is also cultivated according to principles that ensure it contains more vitamins and minerals that non-organically farmed food.

4 Avoid additives. Do not consume food or drink that contains artificial sweeteners, colourings, flavourings or preservatives. This is 'fake' food that the body does not recognise and it therefore becomes toxic.

5 Read the label on packaged foods, and if it lists hydrogenated fats, do not eat it. Trans-fats, the dangerous by-product of the chemical process to create hydrogenated fats, are found in most processed foods yet have been deemed so dangerous that some countries (and, at the time of writing, the city of New York) are banning their use. They are deemed to be carcinogenic (cancer forming) and can promote heart disease.

6 Cut down on meat. If you choose to eat meat then buy the absolute best you can afford by opting for organic. Bacon tends to contain a lot of salt, so be careful to eat it only very occasionally. As an alternative to meat try beans, peas and lentils, and tofu. They are cheap and easy to cook – be inspired by some of the Life Detox recipes.

7 Go alternative for cleaning and gardening. Avoid using conventional household cleaners and opt for natural brands instead (see Suppliers and Further Resources). When you are gardening, avoid the use of pesticides and insecticides.

8 Don't get toxic while making yourself beautiful! Traditional beauty products, such as perfume, nail-varnish remover, make-up, skin care, haircare, hair removal creams and aftershave, all contain potential skin irritants as well as chemicals that can be absorbed through the skin. Instead, choose natural alternatives (see Suppliers and Further Resources) from companies that use non-toxic, organic ingredients. Spray perfume on clothes rather than directly onto the skin, and use aluminium-free deodorant. If you have to have a dental filling, make sure it is porcelain (white) rather than amalgam (silver), which contains mercury, a potentially toxic heavy metal.

9 Try to store foods in glass or ceramic containers rather than plastic or plastic-style wrap. Food can absorb chemicals from the container or wrapping it is stored in. Cooking equipment should be stainless steel or ceramic if possible.

10 Drink more pure water. At the very least, go for a jug filter, but if possible, install a water-purification system in your home.

Bottled water is a good option, but try to buy glass bottles rather than plastic. Carbonated drinks, including water, contain carbon dioxide (CO_2), which often leaches calcium from reserves in the body, so carbonated drinks should be avoided.

11 Take supplements to boost your body's natural detox capability. Specialist detox supplements (see page 68) are the best option for short-term use; however, long-term support can be provided by a good multimineral and vitamin supplement. Psyllium husks (see page 88) help with the removal of toxins.

12 Cook foods lightly Traditional frying creates damaging trans-fats and should be avoided. Browning food through grilling and baking creates harmful free radicals. Try to keep cooking light (as in rapid stir-frying or steaming) and keep roast dinners for special occasions only.

13 Boost your intake of detox nutrients by including a serving of a detox superfood in your diet daily (see page 65). There is a wide range of foods available to suit different tastes and budgets that can be included in meals and snacks with ease.

14 Cut out caffeine, reduce your alcohol and/or nicotine intake. If going 'cold turkey' seems too much then try to reduce your intake little by little each day. Your body will adjust gradually, and, if combined with a nutritious diet, some of the cravings may subside. However, for the Life Detox 7-Day Programme, caffeine and alcohol must be cut out completely for you to enjoy the full benefits.

15 Reduce your mobile phone and television usage. Don't have your mobile phone on charge in your bedroom at night and avoid watching television in bed. Your body does its healing work at night – aim for a 10.30 pm lights-out during detox.

parttwo[2]
the life detox
7-day
programme

chapter seven

Getting Prepared for Your Life Detox

Detoxing need not be hard work, but it does require a bit of forward planning. Life Detox has been designed to be as straightforward as possible, even when you are working. To make things easy on yourself, take a look at our guidelines below to see how best to arrange your week.

When to detox

You can detox at any time of the year, although a change of season, or the month after Christmas, are the most popular times. Detox is a great way to get in shape, physically and mentally, for special occasions such as a wedding, a new job or a holiday, and it can be used to strengthen your immune system by giving your body a rest.

The Life Detox programme is easiest to follow if you start detoxing at a weekend. You can make sure you are prepared for the week ahead by buying as many provisions as possible on the Friday evening and reading through all the detox information at the beginning of Part 2 so that you know what to expect. It is also much better if you have an early night in rather than a late night out prior to beginning your detox journey.

The first couple of days are often the most consuming as you get used to new foods and your body adjusts to living without its habitual toxins. However, by the time Monday morning comes, you will be feeling lighter and brighter, and ready to face the week ahead.

Whenever you choose to detox, you can make the process easier by letting your friends and family know what you are up to (if they will be supportive). Make sure to plan around social engagements so that you are not putting yourself under any extra pressure.

When not to detox

Before you begin your detox check whether you fall into any of the following categories:

☺ If you are pregnant or breastfeeding you should not detox.
☺ If you are taking any medication or having treatment for a specific condition you should talk to your doctor or health practitioner before undertaking the detox programme.
☺ It is not advisable to undertake the mind detox provided in this book if you are on medication for anxiety or depression. If you have been extremely depressed or unable to cope with everyday life or relationships, we recommend you consult your doctor or a professionally trained therapist or counsellor before considering beginning the Life Detox.
☺ If you are feeling unwell or are recovering from a cold or flu, the best course of action is to wait until you feel fully recovered, then begin to detox. However, in the meantime you can start to follow some of the 15 Top Detox Tips in Chapter 6.

Planning your body detox boosters

Take a look at the chart on page 58 so that you can plan for the whole week. We provide optional body boosters each day to help you to enhance your Life Detox results. They support your detox process and you should aim to incorporate as many as possible into your week. The time required for boosters varies from day to day and we have kept the cost as low as possible. It is worth planning your detox week in advance as some boosters, such as massages or saunas, may need to be booked.

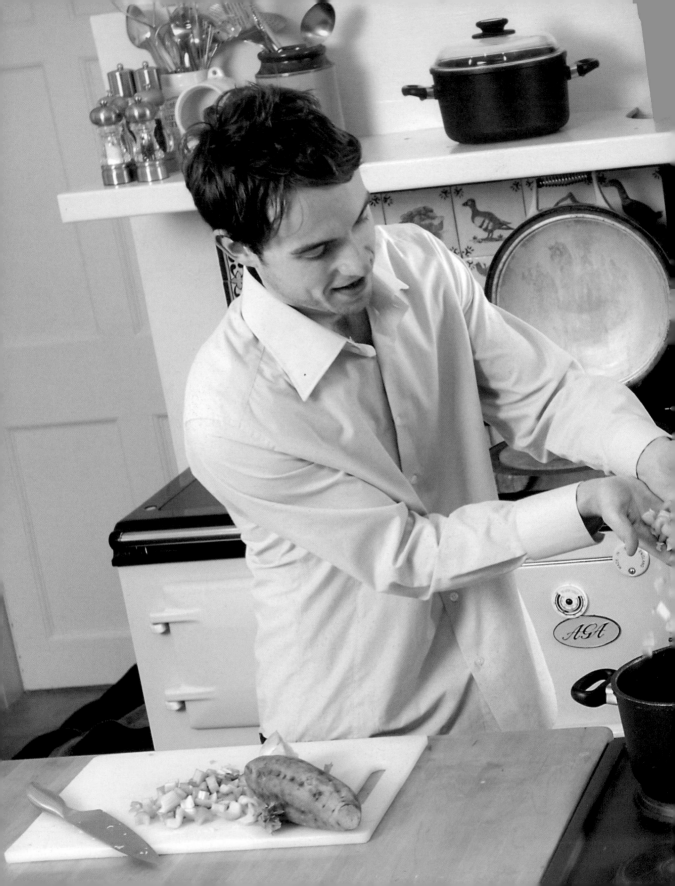

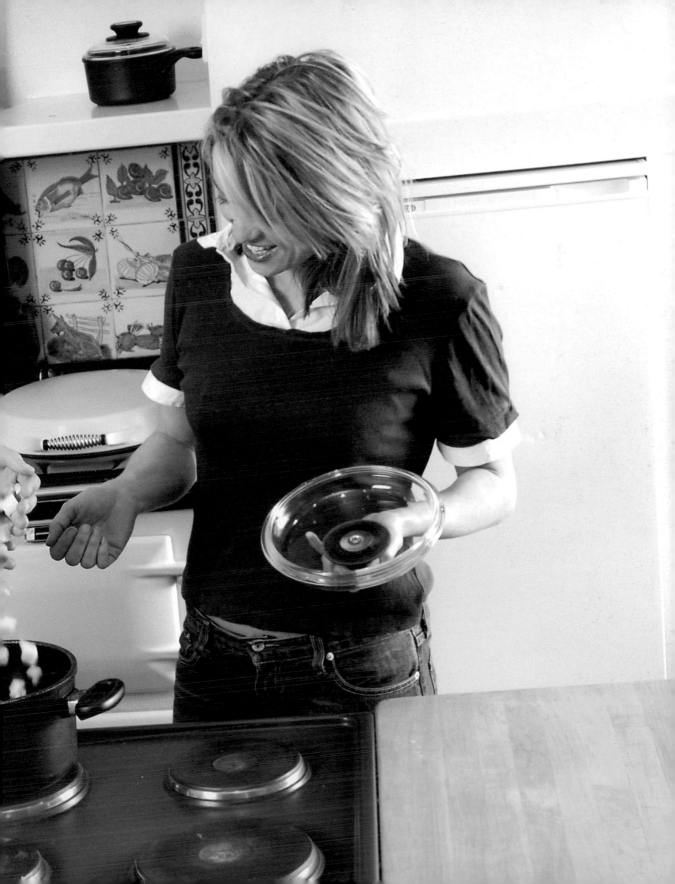

Detox Booster Week Planner

Day	Body booster	Materials, equipment or treatment	Timings
☺ Day 1	30-minute outdoor workout	None	30 minutes
☺ Day 2	Colon cleansing (each day from Day 2 onwards)	Psyllium husks to be added to your juice (available from any health-food shop, or see Suppliers)	2 minutes to prepare
	Herbal teas	Peppermint, dandelion and nettle teas	5 minutes
☺ Day 3	Epsom salts bath	Epsom salts (available from any chemist)	30 minutes
☺ Day 4	Dry skin brushing	Skin brush (see Suppliers)	5 minutes
	Massage	Book at your local therapy centre	30 minutes–1½ hours, depending on treatment
☺ Day 5	Belly breathing and child's pose (yoga)	None, yoga mat if possible	15 minutes
☺ Day 6	Sauna	Book sauna	30 minutes
	Home-made skin care	Ingredients for skin care (see pages 114–115)	1 hour
☺ Day 7	Home hydrotherapy	Shower	1 minute
	Treat yourself: massage/facial/ Epsom salts bath/ yoga/sauna/walk/ horse-riding/cycling/ romantic night in/ colonic hydrotherapy	Depends on treatment	30 minutes–1½ hours, depending on treatment

Shopping for your detox

You will need to buy the following foods and equipment to work through your detox week. Some you'll no doubt already have in your store cupboard. For quantities please look at the programme for each day on pages 79–122 and the recipes on pages 123–141.

Vegetables:
☺ avocados
☺ baby leaf spinach
☺ beetroots
☺ broccoli spears
☺ butternut squash
☺ carrots
☺ celery
☺ chillies, red or green
☺ courgettes
☺ cucumbers
☺ garlic
☺ ginger, fresh root
☺ green vegetables, such as broccoli, kale or green beans
☺ mangetouts
☺ onions, red and white
☺ parsnip (or other root vegetable)
☺ peppers, green, red and yellow
☺ potatoes
☺ radishes
☺ salad leaves, a selection
☺ shallots
☺ spinach
☺ sweet potatoes
☺ tomatoes, including baby plum or cherry tomatoes

Fruit:
☺ apples, dessert and cooking
☺ bananas
☺ blueberries/seasonal berries (frozen or fresh)
☺ grapes
☺ lemons, unwaxed
☺ limes
☺ oranges
☺ papaya
☺ pineapples
☺ strawberries

Fresh produce:
☺ fillet of oily fish, such as salmon
☺ firm white fish or tofu
☺ goat's (feta) or sheep's cheese
☺ natural yogurt or soya yogurt

If you are too busy to make your own hummus or guacamole, add shop-bought tubs (preferably organic) to your shopping list.

Groceries:
☺ almond milk, soya milk or any other non-dairy milk
☺ almonds, flaked
☺ apple cider vinegar
☺ apple juice
☺ apples, dried
☺ apricots, dried
☺ black pepper
☺ butter beans (dried or canned)
☺ cashew nuts
☺ chickpeas (dried or canned)
☺ chilli sauce
☺ coconut, desiccated
☺ coconut milk
☺ eggs, organic
☺ linseed oil
☺ maple syrup
☺ miso soup, minimum 7 sachets (optional, if not making the Detox Broth)
☺ oatcakes
☺ oil
☺ olives
☺ passata (made from puréed and sieved tomatoes)
☺ prunes
☺ quinoa (this is technically a fruit but it looks like a grain and is similar to cous cous)
☺ raisins
☺ rye bread
☺ sea salt
☺ sultanas
☺ Thai green curry paste

☺ vanilla extract
☺ vegetable stock (low-sodium variety or home-made)
☺ walnuts
☺ yeast-free tamari (a wheat-free soy sauce)

Herbs and spices:
(All are optional, but a range will give your food maximum flavour.)
☺ bay leaves
☺ cayenne pepper
☺ chilli flakes
☺ cinnamon
☺ cloves
☺ coriander, fresh
☺ coriander, ground
☺ cumin, ground
☺ kaffir lime leaf
☺ lemon grass
☺ nutmeg
☺ oregano, dried
☺ paprika, ground
☺ parsley, fresh
☺ rosemary, fresh
☺ tarragon, fresh
☺ thyme, fresh
☺ turmeric, ground

Daily juice/smoothie:

You will need a juicer and a blender for this (see Suppliers and Further Resources). However, allowances have been made so that if you don't wish to make these purchases, you can choose a fruit-only option. If you want to juice your own wheatgrass you will need a masticating juicer.

Daily detox booster:

psyllium husks (see Suppliers and Further Resources)

Optional body-booster extras:

500g Epsom salts (available from most chemists)
skin brush (see Suppliers and Further Resources)
yoga mat (see Suppliers and Further Resources)

Go organic

The main way most people accumulate toxins is through processed foods, most of which contains pesticides, preservatives, additives, antibiotics or steroids. Going organic, however, is one of the easiest ways to remove this toxic threat to your health. Organic foods can be found in most supermarkets and health-food shops as well as through internet delivery schemes – try looking online for suppliers.

Does going organic equal going bankrupt?

Cost is currently the biggest argument against buying organic food. However, regularly buying processed foods and drinks and the odd takeaway is more expensive than buying organic food. And, what's more, organic vegetarian cooking can be especially cheap as well as healthy.

Managing detox side effects

A detox works by helping your body get rid of toxins, but remember: these toxins don't just evaporate – they have to be eliminated. You may find yourself on the toilet more than usual; this is a good sign that your body is clearing out. We describe below some of the common side-effects that you might experience during a detox and explain how to combat them. If you want your detox to help with a chronic health problem, whether it is weight gain or a skin problem (see Chapter 4 for a list of conditions detox can help with), then we recommend the detox body boosters alongside the Life Detox programme.

What to look out for during your detox

Here are some quick ways to combat some possible side-effects of the detox, especially during the first few days. If your symptom does not shift, look at Chapter 8 for some superfoods and detox supplements that can give your body a helping hand:

Headaches
The most common side-effect of detoxing is headaches caused by caffeine withdrawal. If possible, cut down your caffeine intake prior to undergoing the detox as it will make the process much easier. If you have a headache:

① Drink plenty of water.
② Stimulate the acupressure points on your temples (in between the outside edge of the eyebrows and the hairline), and rub them with lavender oil.
③ Take an Epsom salts bath (see page 94) and have an early night.
④ Try the yoga 'child's pose' (see page 108) for up to 10 minutes, as long as you feel comfortable.

Unpleasantness in the mouth

If you experience an odd taste in your mouth, a furred tongue or bad breath, try the following:

① Scrape your tongue with a toothbrush or tongue scraper.
② Rinse your mouth out with water and freshly squeezed lemon juice but avoid chewing gum, as this can disrupt your digestion.
③ Take the detox supplements for digestion (see page 77).

Spots or rashes

The skin is the most superficial organ of elimination and sometimes when toxins are moving from deeper areas of the body, the skin shows the effects. This can result in spots, rashes or outbreaks of a previous skin condition. Try not to use commercial spot cream and instead dab a little tea tree oil on the affected area. A rash can be soothed with vitamin E oil direct from a capsule. (Both are available from chemists or health shops.)

Changes in body temperature and sweating

The skin can push its detox powers up a notch during a detox and this should be welcomed. If possible, assist the process with saunas or steam baths, and the situation will improve. If you have had a chronic problem with excess sweating then this will generally improve after the detox.

Side-effects from chronic conditions

Chronic conditions are those that have plagued you for a while, such as IBS, sinusitis, acne or recurring headaches. Acute conditions, however, are those that are happening right now: you have a headache, for example. A detox helps both types. The process of cleansing the body can improve chronic problems and alleviate acute symptoms.

Sometimes, if a chronic problem has been going on for a long time, an acute 'healing crisis' can occur. For example, someone suffering from sinusitis might find that they develop a runny nose during detox, as excess mucus is removed from the body. This kind of acute healing reaction is very helpful and every effort should be made for it to happen naturally, without suppressive medication.

Dealing with toxic emotions

Because your entire body is wired up to feel every emotion, when you detox your body it is normal to feel a little emotional. You may have heard of people laughing or crying for no apparent reason while receiving a body massage. In these cases, the masseuse has hit upon emotionally blocked hotspots – and through their massage has got the emotions flowing again. Something similar can happen when you detox. As you clear physical toxins, you can uncover emotional toxins that may have been stuck in your body for days, weeks, months or even years. If you find that some old emotions begin to surface during your detox, then you can use the exercises and boosters outlined in this book to help you work through and release them for good. This way you will increase your energy levels and reduce any dis-ease that may be occurring in your system.

How to let the toxic emotions go

To clear toxic emotions you simply need to breathe deeply, relax your body and be willing to think about emotionally charged issues in new ways. People tend to tense up their bodies when trying to suppress negative emotions, so if you relax your upper abdominal area just below your chest bone (the area of your body where you process your feelings), you will let your emotions move through your body.

Once your emotions are flowing again you are in the ideal state to tap into your unconscious mind (the part of your mind that generates your emotions) and give it a new way of viewing the perceived problem. This is vital because in order for you to change how you feel about something, you must first change how you think about it. By viewing problematic events and people in more compassionate and optimistic ways, you will no longer make yourself feel bad when you think about them. We provide a mind exercise and detox booster on Day 4 of your Life Detox (see page 104) to help you do this.

chapter eight

Turbocharging Your Life Detox

Your Life Detox 7-Day Programme is a good, basic cleansing detox that will leave you feeling refreshed and vibrant. You can also give it extra power, if you wish, by using some of our suggested body boosters to get the most benefit.

Detox superfoods

One of the easiest ways you can boost your detox is by adding specialist foods into your existing Life Detox diet. 'Superfood' is simply the generic term for something that is especially good for you.

Nature is a storehouse for our detoxing needs. We have followed suit and have classified superfoods according to their natural source. Below is a collection of the most nutrient-rich foods. Choose at least one during the detox week.

Grasses

The grasses listed below contain some of the richest sources of minerals around, but you don't need to head out to a field and start munching; these grasses are most easily digested when they are juiced or in supplement form. Some of them (OK, all of them) don't taste so appetising. However, these foods are just *so good* for you that we urge you not to leave them out. They are densely packed with nutrients, vitamins and minerals that boost immunity – and they help with fat burning, too.

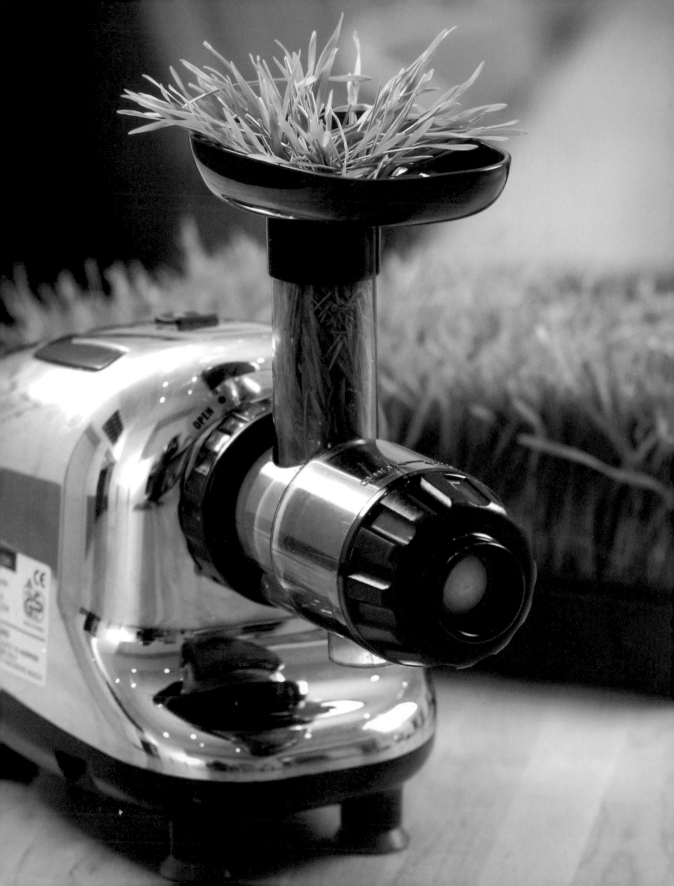

Wheatgrass, barley grass and alfalfa grass If you have a masticating juicer (see page 61), fresh wheatgrass and barley grass can be bought in trays (see Suppliers and Further Resources) and then juiced. You can take it with a strongly flavoured juice to mask its distinctive taste. Alternatively, add a shot of wheatgrass to your favourite juice if you have one at a juice bar.

Powdered or dehydrated wheatgrass, barley grass and alfalfa grass is available in most good health-food shops. A teaspoonful added to juice can make up the nutritional equivalent of two handfuls of broccoli.

Sea superfoods

Some of the most nutritious foods known to man are provided by the sea – a fact not lost on Asian cultures who have been eating seaweed and sea vegetables for centuries (and who have one of the highest life expectancies in the world). Sea vegetables contain virtually all the minerals found in the ocean – the same minerals that are found in human blood. They are an excellent source of iodine and vitamin K and a good source of B vitamins, magnesium, iron and calcium.

Sea vegetables These days, sea vegetables in their dried form can be found in supermarkets. You simply soak them to rehydrate or add to soups when cooking. The most commonly available varieties are nori, wakame, dulse and kelp. Add a tablespoon of dried seaweed to your soup for the duration of your 7-Day detox.

Spirulina, chloerella and blue-green algae If you don't like the thought of eating seaweed you can try supplementing with algae. Don't worry, there is no need to scrape the bottom of your neighbour's pond – the health-giving algae come in liquid, powder or tablet form. An excellent source of protein, algae can boost immunity, improve mental performance and are an excellent all-round source of vitamins, minerals and hard-to-get amino acids.

Sprouts

Not Brussels sprouts but fast-growing, young, green plants. The sprouting phase of growing plants contains a power-packed energy high. 'Sprout', therefore, describes the phase at which you eat the plant, rather than the variety. However, some plants are more commonly sprouted than others: alfalfa and mung beans are frequently found in the chill cabinet in health-food shops and supermarkets.

Aim to use a small handful of sprouts each day – adding them to stir-fries and salads.

Healing plants

At our detox clinics we work alongside a medical herbalist and have come to learn and love the power of herbs and healing plants. Here are our favourites specifically for detoxing:

Aloe vera can speed up the alkalising process in the body and soothe the gut lining. Excellent if you have ever suffered from digestive complaints. Take in liquid form mixed with a fresh juice.
Echinacea This magical herb is found everywhere now, due to its incredible rise in popularity in recent years. It is best known for its immune-boosting effect but it is also great for boosting the lymphatic system. Take in liquid or capsule form. Like many herbs, echinacea works best when taken periodically rather than continually. Finish one course of tablets or tincture, have a break for a month, then start again.

Detox supplements

We recommend using specialist detox supplements only. The supplements listed below are balanced nutritionally and biochemically to aid the detox process, while supporting your body's needs. There is no need to take any other nutritional supplements during the 7-day detox as these formulae are designed to cover everything you need. Choose at least one from the following list.

Liver support

The first vital step for the majority of people to take is to support the liver, as this is the main organ of detoxification. Detox Support Formula is a specialist formula designed specifically for this purpose (see Suppliers and Further Resources). It is a gentle yet effective way to heal the body from the inside out.

Take two tablets daily for a gentle start, or, if you are ready for a powerful detox, then go straight into four tablets a day.

Digestion support

For all-round good health during and after detoxing, we suggest Colon Support Formula, a fantastic blend of herbs, spices and natural cleansing agents that gently assists your digestive tract. This supplement is very powerful in combination with psyllium (see page 96) but in itself can provide longer-term support if you want to continue detoxing or have had problems with a sluggish bowel or IBS symptoms in the past.

Take two tablets daily for a gentle start, or four tablets daily for the duration of the Life Detox if you want a stronger detox.

Home detox kit

If you wish to take your detox a step further, you can use a combined approach that supports the organs of elimination and detoxification at a cellular level. However, as the detox requirements are complex and difficult to source for many people, Amanda has worked on creating an easy-to-use kit for a 7- or 14-day home detox (see Suppliers and Further Resources). The kit includes:

☺ **Colon Support Formula** (see above)
☺ **Detox Support Formula** (see above)
☺ **A probiotic bacteria** designed to help promote beneficial bacteria in the gut.
☺ **Bentonite clay** A formula used to help remove toxic heavy metals from the body.

☺ **Skin brush** A natural vegetable-bristle brush used to enhance lymphatic drainage and assist in the breakdown of cellulite.

☺ **A guide to detoxing**

Other ways to boost your detox

To help the body eliminate toxins and to give you an all-round cleanse, you could try the following suggestions.

Colon cleansing

Although not the most glamorous of detox tools, colon cleansing is certainly one of the most effective. Supporting the elimination of toxins by assisting the bowel to expel them (using an enema) is a technique that has been around for centuries – it is perfectly safe and comfortable. Many people opt for colonic hydrotherapy (see Suppliers and Further Resources), which has a powerful cleansing effect. Enemas can also be used at less cost but need to be administered at home under the guidance of a nutritionist or naturopath. Check out the section on colon cleansing on our website for more information (www.lifedetox.co.uk).

Complementary therapies

All complementary therapies – such as massage, acupuncture and reflexology – work on balancing energy. They will enhance your Life Detox programme, so do try to make time in your schedule to organise an appointment for yourself. The most important aspect of choosing a complementary therapy to support your detox process is that you enjoy the experience. Find out about the ones that appeal to you – it truly is a personal choice.

If you do not know of any complementary therapists in your area, type the therapy you are most interested in into an Internet search engine to find the national association (see page 156 for a selection). You will then find directory listings of practitioners throughout the country.

chapter nine

Exercise During Your Detox

No detoxification programme is complete without considering exercise. Humans are supposed to be energetic by nature – our bodies are made for moving. In fact, in many traditions, disease is thought of simply as a manifestation of blocked chi (or life force), or energy. Therapies such as acupuncture are based on unblocking the trapped chi and letting it flow again.

During the Life Detox we urge you to get your own energy moving. It's not just about the hidden force of chi, it's also because an active body helps your system to detox, and it boosts endorphins, keeping you feeling positive and balanced. Getting the body moving assists the cleansing process and helps you to boost your metabolism in the long run.

Daily body exercise

For the week-long programme, the minimum daily exercise is a 15-minute workout. We have provided full instructions on our favourite detox exercise, which is yoga, but have given skipping or rebounding (see page 74) as an alternative indoor workout. However, if you are already a regular exerciser, please feel free to incorporate either the yoga or other options into your existing programme.

☺

Exercise: 15-minute yoga workout

One of the best exercises for assisting your body's cleansing is yoga. The positions through which the body moves during the practice of yoga help to massage the organs of elimination and increase oxygenation of the tissues. Yoga works on balancing the mind and the body in an incredibly powerful way. Don't worry if you feel you are inflexible or are a complete beginner – this simple sequence of yoga postures, called *Surya Namaskar* or Sun Salutation, are 12 postures performed in a single, graceful flow. Traditionally, it is performed at dawn, facing the rising sun, and it is most effective as a sequence used to begin the day. It limbers up the whole body and gets the energy flowing. Even if you manage just one sequence you will feel the difference.

Yoga should be practised in silence because the rhythm of the breath is important. In other words, no television or radio noises in the background! Each movement is coordinated with the breath. Inhale as you extend or stretch, and exhale as you fold or contract.

Try the Sun Salutation series opposite, to add a range of stretching postures to your detox. A single round of the series consists of two complete sequences: one for the right side of the body and the other for the left. One complete round takes approximately 3–4 minutes so aim to do at least two rounds every morning.

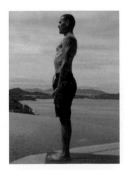

1 Exhale and stand tall.

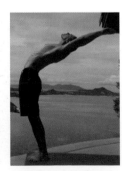

2 Inhale and sweep your hands above your head.

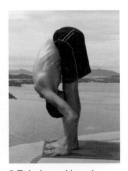

3 Exhale and bend forward with your head towards your shins.

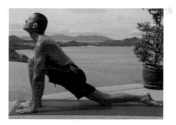

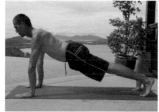

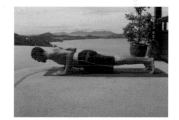

4 Inhale and step your right leg back into a deep lunge.

5 Exhale and step your left leg back into the plank position. Hold in position. Inhale and pull your tummy in.

6 Inhale and bend your arms into a press-up position, keeping your elbows in close to your body. (You can have your knees on the floor if you wish.)

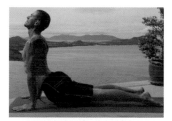

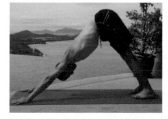

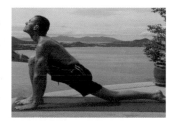

7 Inhale and stretch forwards and up, arching your back. Use your arms to lift your torso as far as feels comfortable. Keep your shoulders down. Your hands should be in front of your hips. Look upwards.

8 Exhale and tuck your toes under. Lift your bottom back, and press back into an upside-down V shape.

9 Inhale and step your right foot forwards between your hands and knees. Exhale and do the same with the left foot.

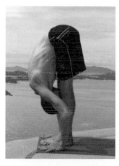

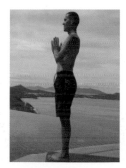

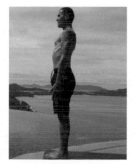

10 On the same exhale, bring your feet together and straighten your legs, head to shins.

11 Inhale, stand up slowly and return to your starting position.

12 Repeat the series, starting with your left leg.

Exercise: 15-minute indoor workout

Skip or rebound for 15 minutes each detox day at a time that suits you. This kick-start is a great way to boost lymphatic drainage and get a quick but effective workout.

Skipping requires no introduction, as most of us have skipped as children, but it really is good exercise. Lightweight ropes are much easier to handle than the heavy rope variety. Make sure you wear supportive footwear.

Rebounding (jumping on a mini-trampoline) is a fun and safe way to increase fitness. Vigorous exercise such as rebounding is reported to increase lymph flow by 15 to 30 times, depending on how high you bounce. This lymphatic stimulation is of great help to the detox process. (See Suppliers and Further Resources for rebounder trampolines.)

Optional body booster

On Day 1 we also suggest an optional 30-minute exercise body booster to kick-start your detox. However, if you're feeling full of energy and enthusiasm, we highly recommend taking this exercise each day – you'll certainly feel the benefit.

Exercise: 30-minute outdoor workout

For your 30-minute workout, try a brisk walk or light jog. You should work up a light sweat but still be able to hold a conversation while you walk or jog. If you like to escape to some music then use an MP3 player with upbeat tracks that will help keep your pace brisk.

Get moving

Help to get the maximum benefit from your detox by taking some other daily exercise. Sometimes a bit of imagination is needed to find time to fit exercising into your day, especially if you are sitting down in an office all day or have a hectic day with young children – but it's amazing how fit you can get by going out for a walk during your lunch hour at work or, if you have small children, pushing a buggy up and down a hill for 30 minutes a day! Find ways that will suit your own circumstances; here are a few ideas to give you some inspiration:

☺ Walk to work instead of driving or using public transport.
☺ Take the stairs instead of the lift.
☺ Walk off your lunch or dinner – head outdoors after eating and assist your digestion in the process.
☺ Pick up groceries at a local store rather than an out-of-town supermarket, and walk there and back (take a backpack for carrying items home).
☺ Walk the dog – or borrow a dog! Most people are delighted if you offer to help walk their pet pooch.

Once you get into the routine of moving about more during your day it will become a habit and you will feel much fitter and happier as a result.

☺

chapter ten

The Life Detox 7-Day Programme

Each day of your Life Detox has a theme for the body and another for the mind. The themes take you one step at a time on your detox journey, helping you to transform your body, mind and life in seven days. The different themes are explained in more detail as they appear, and each day comes with tasks, exercises and optional detox boosters to help you to clear physical, mental and emotional toxins. The themes will be as follows:

Day 1: Saturday
For the body: Detox To-do List
For the mind: Toxic To-do List

Day 2: Sunday
For the body: Clean Your Core
For the mind: Clean Your Habits

Day 3: Monday
For the body: Detox Your Liver
For the mind: Detox Your Thoughts

Day 4: Tuesday
For the body: Let Life Flow
For the mind: Toxic Emotions Go!

Day 5: Wednesday
For the body: Boost Your Breathing
For the mind: Boost Your Self-image

Day 6: Thursday
For the body: Shape up the Skin
For the mind: Sort out the Stress

Day 7: Friday
For the body: Energise Your Body
For the mind: Energise Your Mind

Have a journal that you can use during your detox week to note down anything you need to remember as you go through the programme and to use for your goodnight questions, which we explain below.

Understanding the Life Detox schedule

The Life Detox 7-Day Programme is designed to be followed while working a 9.00 am to 6.00 pm day. If you do not work or are on holiday while doing your Life Detox, then you can use the extra time to explore the optional detox boosters (there is one for the body and one for the mind each day). To ensure it is easy to follow, the Life Detox schedule is similar each day.

Morning (before 9.00 am)

☺ Warm-start drink (2 slices of lemon or lime in hot water).
☺ Power-up Process. The Power-up Process helps to you start your day with energy and mental alertness. Please aim to do it within 30 minutes of waking.
☺ Yoga workout or skipping/rebounding.
☺ Morning juice, smoothie or fruit.

Daytime (between 9.00 am and 6.00 pm)

☺ Mid-morning raw-power snack.
☺ Liver-loving lunch.
☺ Afternoon pick-me-up.
☺ Daytime mind detoxer (exercise). Your daytime task (between 9.00 am and 6.00 pm if possible) is to clear one, two or three items from the Toxic To-do List that you will prepare on Day 1 (depending on the time and effort involved for each item).

Evening (between 6.00 pm and 10.00 pm)

☺ Detox dinner.

☺ Optional body booster.

☺ Evening mind detoxer (exercise). The mind detox tasks happen during the evenings. Allow anything from 15 to 45 minutes in total for the tasks, depending upon how involved
you want to become.

☺ Optional mind boosters. These are provided each day to help you boost your Life Detox results.

Just before bed (any time between 10.00 pm and 10.30 pm)

☺ Goodnight journal questions. Night-time journal-writing during your detox is useful, as it can be a time of great mental clarity, creativity and learning. Writing just before bed is also an effective way to quieten your mind.

You are now ready to start on Day 1 of your Life Detox.

dayone saturday

Congratulations! By embarking on this 7-Day Life Detox you are taking a massive step towards supreme health and happiness. Today you will organise yourself and get clear about the results you want from your detox week.

LifeDetox daily schedule

Upon rising 2 slices of lemon or lime in hot water

Morning mind detoxer Power-up Process

Daily body exercise Yoga workout or skipping/rebounding (page 82)

Jump-out-of-bed juice Go Go Juice, or fruit

Mid-morning raw-power snack Delicious Dip

Liver-loving lunch Tomato and Bean Soup (page 130), plus one of the following options: 4 oatcakes, 4 rice cakes or 2 slices of rye bread (or other non-wheat bread)

Afternoon pick-me-up A small handful of nuts and seeds (page 126)

Daytime mind detoxer Write Toxic To-do List and Life Detox Results

Detox two-course dinner First course: Detox Salad (page 130); main course: Chilli con Veggie (page 128)

Optional body booster (exercise) 30-minute outdoor workout (page 74)

Just before bed Goodnight questions

For the body: Detox To-do List

Body detox daily update

Today is all about getting ready for your detox week. If you haven't done so already, make sure you have all the ingredients necessary for the next few days' meals and juices. If you are aiming for weight loss, stand on the scales first thing this morning and make a note in your journal. Avoid using the scales again until the morning after your detox is complete.

At this early stage of detox, you need to boost your intake of antioxidants so that they can start neutralising the toxins. Antioxidants help to prevent cell and tissue damage and are used in the fight against disease. Vitamins C and E are two of the best-known antioxidants and they are abundant in organic fruit and vegetables (see our Go Go Juice and vegetables for dipping). Make sure you are following the Life Detox diet fully and that your intake of fruit and vegetables is high.

Today's juice: Go Go Juice

Put ½ pineapple (peeled), 2 apples (cored), 4 carrots (scrubbed) and 1 orange (peeled) through the juicer (see page 124).

Fast facts about Go Go Juice

This is a delicious combination that is a great kick-start to your detox week. All the ingredients work on helping your body to eliminate toxins while boosting your daily vitamin intake. It is also a high-energy drink with a pleasant, sweet taste – a gentle way to break you into the juicing lifestyle. Pineapple helps to reduce inflammation and can help with congestion problems, making it ideal as the key ingredient of this juice. Carrots and apples are a mainstay of detox drinks because they aid the detoxing process and boost antioxidants, while oranges are high in vitamin C. Enjoy!

Delicious Dip

For your mid-morning raw-power snack, choose a handful of vegetable sticks (pepper, carrot, courgette, cucumber, celery), or a piece of fruit of your choice and dip into 1–2 tbsp Raw Hummus or Guacamole (page 125).

Fluids

Keeping your fluids up is essential during detox. Throughout each day, consume no less than four 225ml (8fl oz) glasses of water.

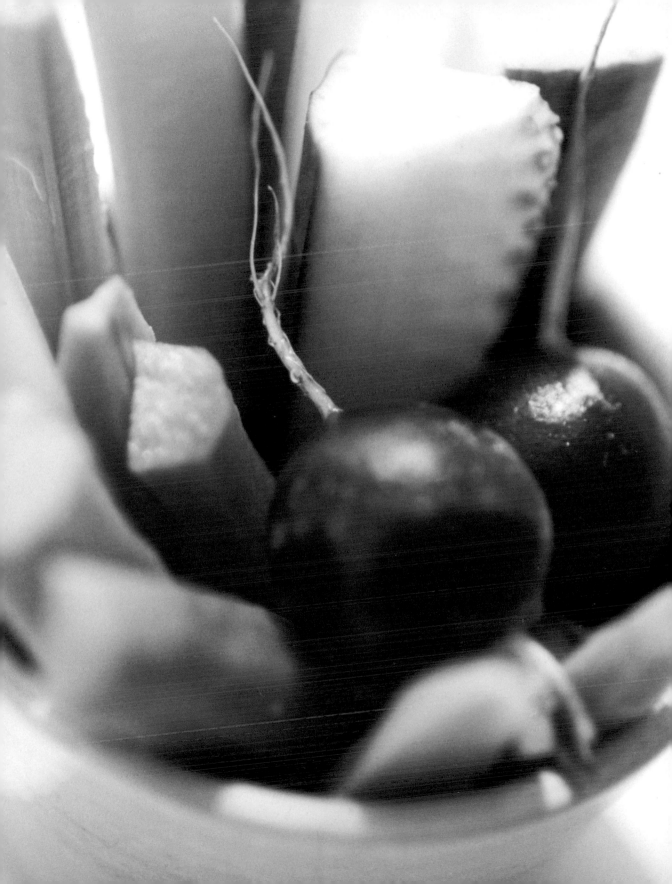

The following can also be taken each day:
☺ Unlimited herbal tea
☺ Unlimited Life Detox Broth (see page 127)
☺ Two sachet servings of miso soup (see page 127)

Added extras

As well as the snacks and meals listed in your daily schedule, you can have the following each day:
☺ 2 tbsp olive oil (for cooking or for a salad dressing)
☺ 1 tsp butter (for spreading)
☺ 2 tbsp linseed (flax) oil (for a salad dressing or in smoothies)

Body exercise

Include your minimum 15-minute yoga, skipping or rebounding workout (or your existing exercise programme) as described in Chapter 9 (page 74).

Optional body booster (exercise)

To kick-start your detox week the 30-minute outdoor workout (see page 74) couldn't be better. You could also include it in Days 2 to 6 if you want to turbocharge your detox (see Chapter 8).

For the mind: Toxic To-do List

Mind detox daily update

The purpose of today's mind detox is to help you become clear about what you want to achieve from your life detox experience.

Morning mind detoxer

Do this Power-up Process each morning as part of your daily detox schedule.

Power-up Process (time: 5 minutes)

① Stand with your legs shoulder-width apart, and your knees slightly bent. With pelvis tucked forward, let your shoulders drop down, relax your jaw and close your eyes.
② Imagine placing a warm smile on the top of your head and let it melt down over the front of your face, neck, chest, and the entire front of your body to your feet and back into the earth.
③ Imagine placing another warm smile on the top of your head and this time imagine it melting down the back of your head, neck, back and all the way down into the earth.
④ Imagine placing a third warm smile on the top of your head, and

this time let it melt through your head (relaxing your mind), down through your centre and back into the earth.

⑤ Now imagine roots coming out from the soles and heels of your feet, going deep into the earth and directly below you and spreading out as far as the earth's core. This is how it feels to be grounded.

⑥ Imagine golden and warm energy coming up through the roots and entering into your body through your feet as you breathe deeply and slowly. Inhale and imagine pulling the energy up through your body and over the top of your head. Exhale and let it all go down over your face and the front of your body, returning to the earth. Repeat step 6 a further five times.

Daytime mind detoxer

Take your time over writing your Toxic To-do List because working through and clearing the items off it forms the basis of your daytime activities over the next seven days. If you stick to clearing at least one, two or three items from your Toxic To-do List each day, you will be able to clear between seven and 21 toxic items in just seven days – transforming your life and making you feel great.

Once you've written your Toxic To-do List you will be much clearer on what you want to get from your

Life Detox experience. You can add to your list during the detox week if more toxic items come to mind.

Top Tip
Keep your Life Detox goals, theme and symbol (see page 93) at the forefront of your mind this week. Remember that your unconscious mind is always helping you to move towards and become whatever you are focusing on the most. So by focusing on what you want from your Life Detox, you will be assisting your unconscious mind to help you obtain it.

Write Toxic To-do List (time: 5 – 10 minutes)

For your Toxic To-do List, in your journal write down all the things that you would benefit from cleaning, fixing, organising and resolving. Include those things you've been meaning to do for a while but haven't got round to, and the stuff you have been putting off. It may be paying an outstanding bill, cleaning a cupboard or organising a dental appointment. You can use the following headings to help you:

☺ My health
☺ My relationships
☺ My work
☺ My finances
☺ Disorganisation and messes

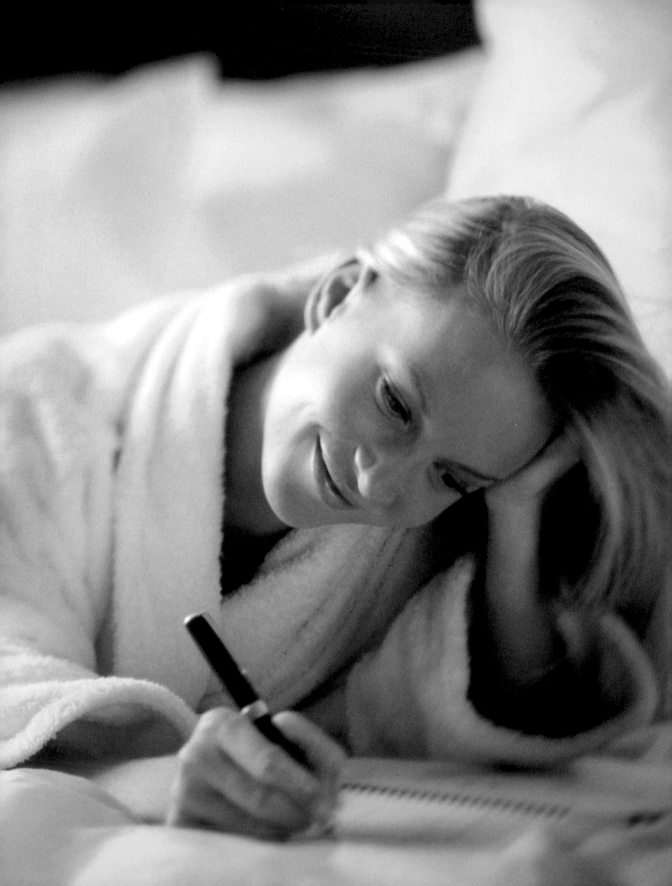

☺ Bad habits
☺ Toxic environment
☺ Toxic emotions

Life Detox Results (time: 5–10 minutes)
Work through the following to find your Life Detox goals, theme and symbol.

Goals
Answer the following questions in your journal:
① What do I want to gain from my Life Detox?
(You might want more confidence, enhanced energy or healthier-looking skin.)
② What do I want to let go of during my Life Detox?
(You may want to let go of excess weight, put a stop to your IBS, no longer feel angry about past events or break a bad habit such as smoking.)
③ How will I know I have achieved the above results?
(List the evidence, such as 'I will be able to enjoy a night out without smoking' or 'I will be able to fit into my favourite pair of jeans'.)

Theme
If you could summarise what you want from your Life Detox in just *one* positive word, what would it be? For example, if you want to lose weight, make sure the word you choose creates an image of a 'slimmer, healthier you' in your mind's eye. Write it in your journal. This is your theme for your Life Detox. Hold it in your mind throughout the week.

Symbol
Relax your body and let your mind rest on your detox goals and theme. Now draw a symbol that you will be able to hold in your mind and which encompasses your intention.

Goodnight journal questions
Each night before bed, please answer the following questions in your journal:
① What was the best part of my day?
(Take a moment to feel gratitude.)
② What have I done today to clear physical and emotional toxins from my body and life?
③ Why should I continue my Life Detox journey tomorrow?

daytwosunday

Today focuses on helping you get your digestion working efficiently. You also have the opportunity to break some toxic habits and use the next few days to build new ones that make you healthier and happier.

LifeDetox daily schedule

Upon rising 2 slices of lemon or lime in hot water

Morning mind detoxer Power-up Process (page 82)

Daily body exercise Yoga workout or skipping/rebounding (page 74)

Jump-out-of-bed smoothie Digestive Delight Smoothie, or fruit

Mid-morning raw-power snack Delicious Dip

Liver-loving lunch Leftover Chilli con Veggie from Day 1, plus one of the following options: 4 oatcakes, 4 rice cakes or 2 slices of rye bread (or other non-wheat bread)

Afternoon pick-me-up Mug of Life Detox Broth (page 127), or sachet of miso soup

Daytime mind detoxer Remove one to three items from your Toxic To-do List

Detox three-course dinner First course: small bowl of leftover Tomato and Bean Soup from Day 1 (200ml/7fl oz/⅓ pint); main course: Warm Butternut, Spinach and Roasted Goat's Cheese Salad (page 131); dessert: Stewed Apples with Blueberries (page 131) or Compote (page 132)

Optional body booster Herbal teas

Evening mind detoxer Clean Your Habits

Optional mind booster New Habit Generator

Just before bed Goodnight questions

For the body: Clean Your Core

Body detox daily update

If you have chosen to follow our 'when to detox' guidelines then you will be following Day 2 on a Sunday. In order to make the transition from the weekend to the working week, tonight you are allowed to choose one of our dreamy desserts!

Remember, it's what you absorb from your food that matters. No matter how much you may cleanse other areas of the body, if you do not clean out the digestive tract, the very toxins you are working so hard to get rid of elsewhere may still be circulated throughout the body. Think of your digestion as an internal sewer system – if it gets clogged up then a range of harmful toxins can build up.

First signs

Your digestion feels the impact of detox straight away, beginning with your mouth. If you have woken up with whitish or yellowish residue on your tongue then your digestive system is beginning to clear out. Use a tongue scraper or the back of a small spoon to remove this mucous film – not just today but every morning of the detox.

You may also experience all kinds of weird and wonderful noises from the depths of your body when your diet first changes. The important thing is not to worry; it is not a bad sign, just your body adjusting. Follow the tips below and it should soon calm down:

① Make sure you chew food properly and don't drink while eating (drink water before and after your meals).

② Eat only when relaxed and comfortable; eating when stressed stops the digestion from working efficiently and can result in wind, indigestion or heartburn.

③ Use psyllium husks (see page 88).

If our detox diet is very different from your usual diet then there is a high chance you are experiencing cravings for your 'normal' foods or for addictive substances such as caffeine. Any withdrawal symptoms will mark a temporary phase only, so power through it (see the Power-up Process). If you need help with breaking bad habits, jump ahead and use Sandy's mind techniques Detox Your Thoughts, and Coming to New Conclusions on pages 96–97.

Today's smoothie: Digestive Delight Smoothie

Juice ½ pineapple (peeled), 2 apples (cored) and a small handful of strawberries (hulled and stalks removed). Put the juice in a blender with ½ papaya (peeled and seeded). Add one teaspoon of psyllium husks stirred quickly into the smoothie and follow with one 225ml (8fl oz) glass of water.

Optional body booster: herbal teas

A pleasant way to give the digestion a boost is to brew up a special digestive detox tea, which can be taken hot, warm or cold throughout the day. This special blend contains herbs that boost digestion and elimination, as well as providing support for your other organs of elimination. Single organic tea bags are best, as pre-blended tea bags can contain flavourings. Place one of each of the tea bags in a teapot and sip throughout the day.

Peppermint Soothing on the digestive system, calming, refreshing and deals with bloating, as it calms down the whole of the lower colon.

Dandelion Supports the whole system of elimination through the bowel and bladder, as well as assisting the liver.

Nettle Encourages the elimination of acid from the body, especially uric acid (one of the acids that can form in the joints). It also contains traces of essential minerals and iron.

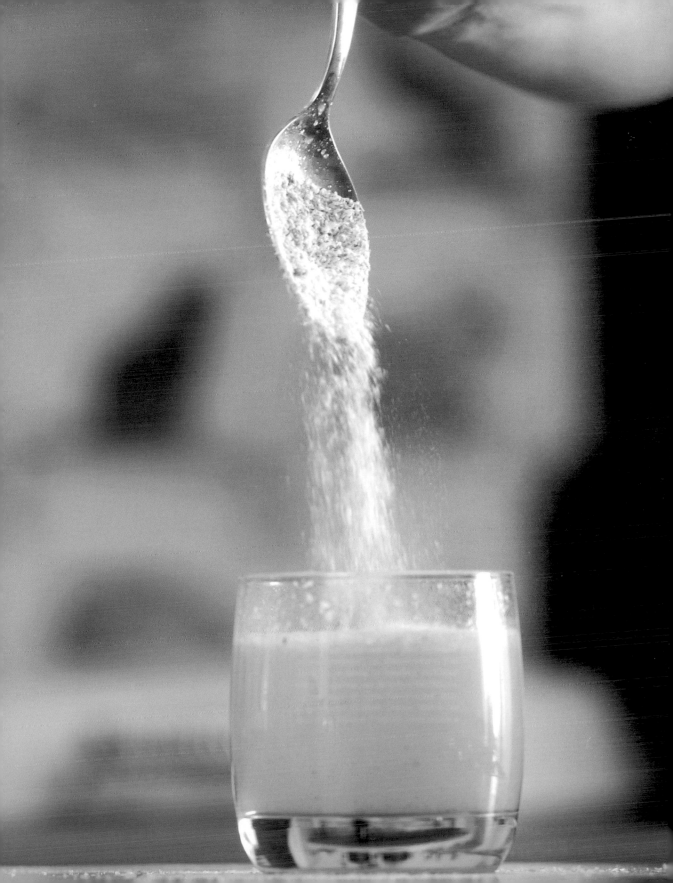

Delicious Dip

For your mid-morning raw-power snack, choose a handful of vegetable sticks (pepper, carrot, courgette, cucumber, celery), or a piece of fruit of your choice and dip into 1–2 tbsp Raw Hummus or Guacamole (page 125).

Fluids and added extras

Remember to drink plenty of fluids and include your added extras as you did on Day 1 (page 79).

Body exercise

Include your minimum 15-minute yoga, skipping or rebounding workout (or your existing exercise programme) as described in Chapter 9 (page 74).

For the mind: Clean Your Habits

Mind detox daily update

We all have habits. Some are helpful for our health and happiness, whereas others are toxic. Do you have habits that you wish you could break? Well, today's the day you let go of them for good – see our Evening Mind Detoxer.

Morning mind detoxer

Practise the Power-up Process from Day 1 when you first rise (page 82).

Daytime mind detoxer

Look at your Toxic To-do List from Day 1 (page 82) and deal with between one and three items so that they can be removed from the list.

Evening mind detoxer

Have you ever tried to break a habit, but keep doing it, despite knowing it's bad for you? This is why: most people try to break a bad habit by focusing on the habit they don't want. This creates a picture in the mind's eye of the unwanted behaviour, which is then interpreted by your unconscious mind as a direct order. The result is you continuing with the familiar, old habit.

Clean Your Habits (time: 5 minutes per habit)
In your journal, re-create the headings and blank rows from the table opposite. In the first row, write the toxic habit that you want to stop. In the row beneath, get clear on how you've been benefiting from the bad

Clean Your Habits (example)

Old toxic habit	Watching TV every night.
Benefits of the bad habit	Helps me relax after a stressful day.
New helpful habit	Going for a run twice a week.
Why build the new habit?	Fresh air, improve fitness, healthier heart, lungs, etc., fun, sociable when running with friend, live life instead of watching someone else live theirs on TV!
First steps	Dust off my running shoes or get new ones; call friend to see which night this week he/she is free; decide a route; set a date and stick to it – rain, hail or shine!

habit. Then decide on the new helpful habit you want to build instead, and list its benefits (make sure they are compelling and motivational). Now, write down the first steps you are going to make to build the new habit, and commit yourself to a specific date or time to get started.

It takes around 21 days to build a new habit. If you make the commitment that you will never quit, then success becomes inevitable. A genuine commitment allows for no excuses. It makes breaking bad habits inevitable because you focus on the benefits and efforts of the new habits rather than the problems with the old ones. Here is a powerful detox booster:

Optional mind booster

New Habit Generator (time: 5 minutes)

Use this detox booster to install any helpful habits that you want. You've probably heard of the power of visualisation (creating a positive picture in your mind). You can get even better results if you combine a visual image with positive feelings. Sandy calls it 'feelingisation'. You then send an even more powerful message to your unconscious mind, which it duly follows.

① Relax your body and mind completely for up to 1 minute. If your 'feelingisation' is going to involve you getting animated, then you will probably need to stand, so keep your eyes open. If it is more peaceful, you may wish to sit.

② Now enjoy your future for up to 3 minutes. Do this by visualising yourself enjoying all the benefits of having the helpful habit and feeling how great you would feel. See yourself in the picture and tune into all of the positive feelings associated with the new habit.

③ Spend 1 minute appreciating the efforts you've made to build the new helpful habit. Give yourself a well-deserved pat on the back. Your unconscious mind is designed to choose the options in life that are the safest and easiest for you. Linking the visual image of the habit in your mind with positive feelings encourages your unconscious mind to install it as a habit.

④ You can use this process throughout your Life Detox week (and beyond if you wish).

Your detox results
Look at the Life Detox goals and theme that you wrote down on Day 1 (page 86) and make sure you are taking steps to help yourself achieve them.

Goodnight journal questions

Answer the following questions in your journal:

① What was the best part of my day? (Take a moment to feel gratitude.)

② What have I done today to clear physical and emotional toxins from my body and life?

③ Why should I continue my Life Detox journey tomorrow?

daythreemonday

Your liver is the main organ of detoxification, and your detox today concentrates on helping it to perform better. You also work on cleaning your mind of any toxic thoughts that may be negatively affecting your body and life.

LifeDetox daily schedule

Upon rising 2 slices of lemon or lime in hot water

Morning mind detoxer Power-up Process (page 82)

Daily body exercise Yoga workout or skipping/rebounding (page 74)

Jump-out-of-bed smoothie Ultimate Liver Lover, or fruit

Mid-morning raw-power snack Delicious Dip

Liver-loving two-course lunch Butternut and Carrot Soup (page 141), plus one of the following options: 4 oatcakes, 4 rice cakes or 2 slices of rye bread (or other non-wheat bread); plus Stewed Apples with Blueberries or Compote left over from Day 2

Afternoon pick-me-up A small handful of nuts and seeds (page 126)

Daytime mind detoxer Remove one to three items from your Toxic To-do List

Detox two-course dinner First course: mug (200ml/7fl oz/⅓ pint) of Butternut and Carrot Soup left over from lunchtime; main course: Baked Fish with Rosemary Roasted Veggies (page 134)

Optional body booster Epsom salts bath

Evening mind detoxer Detox Your Thoughts

Optional mind booster Coming to New Conclusions

Just before bed Goodnight questions

For the body: Detox Your Liver

Body detox daily update

By day three your system is really beginning to work hard at detoxing – so today's aim is to be easy on yourself and, if possible, take things at a more relaxed pace. The three organs that represent the powerhouse of detoxification (including fat metabolism and water balance) are the liver, gallbladder and kidneys. Many people need some help to boost their liver function, which can be compromised by excess alcohol, caffeine, chemicals and fatty foods, and insufficient mineral-rich foods such as nuts and seeds. Anyone on medication can also be putting extra stress on their liver. The liver is also related to stored emotions. We strongly recommend you make time for the mind detox today, which will be complemented by today's relaxing body booster.

Today's smoothie: Ultimate Liver Lover

Blend together 1 lemon (peeled), a small piece of fresh root ginger (peeled and finely chopped), 2 apples (cored), 3 oranges (peeled) and ½ banana.

Add one teaspoon of psyllium husks stirred quickly into the smoothie and follow with one 225ml (8fl oz) glass of water.

Fast facts about Ultimate Liver Lover
The citrus fruits lemon and orange makes this smoothie the ultimate liver lover because both are packed with vitamin C, which helps liver functioning. Lemons also contain a compound called limonene, which acts as a stimulant for the gallbladder, and this in turn also helps boost the liver. Apples add a powerful detox kick and ginger helps reduce inflammation, boosts circulation and calms the gut, as well as giving the smoothie a refreshing taste. The banana is a good source of potassium and vitamin B_6 and is a great mood enhancer due to its levels of tryptophan, which the body converts to serotonin, the ultimate 'feel good' hormone.

Delicious Dip

For your mid-morning raw-power snack, choose a handful of vegetable sticks (pepper, carrot, courgette, cucumber, celery), or a piece of fruit of your choice and dip into 1–2 tbsp Raw Hummus or Guacamole (page 125).

Fluids and added extras

Remember to drink plenty of fluids and include your added extras as you did on Day 1 (page 79).

Body exercise

Include your minimum 15-minute yoga, skipping or rebounding workout (or your existing exercise programme) as described in Chapter 9 (page 74).

Optional body boosters:

Epsom salts bath (time: about 20 minutes)
Detoxing needn't be hard work. Relaxing in a lovely warm bath of Epsom salts will help to draw out toxins from the blood and to also take the stress away from the liver and kidneys. Epsom salts are magnesium sulphate, a naturally occurring mineral that has been used since the 17th century for purging and healing. Bathing in the salts allows your skin to absorb the beneficial magnesium while drawing out toxins from your body. You can enhance the experience by lighting candles and listening to relaxing music. Add about 500g (1lb 2oz) of Epsom salts to comfortably warm bath water and soak yourself for about 20 minutes. Do not use soap, as it will interfere with the action of the salts. Try to keep warm and rest for at least one hour afterwards. (Epsom salts can be bought at minimum cost from any chemist.)

Caution **If you have high blood pressure or a heart condition, you should not have an Epsom salts bath. If you have any joint pain, use only about 100g (3$^{1}/_{2}$oz).**

For the mind: Detox Your Thoughts

Mind detox daily update

Today is your opportunity to become aware of your toxic thoughts and to come to some new and helpful conclusions about yourself, other people and the world you live in. We tell you how in our Evening Mind Detoxer below.

Morning mind detoxer

Practise the Power-up Process from Day 1 when you first rise (page 82).

Daytime mind detoxer

Look at your Toxic To-do List from Day 1 (page 82) and deal with between one and three items so that they can be removed from the list.

Evening mind detoxer

Your thoughts affect every cell in your body, so you can change your body by cleaning your mind of the toxic thoughts. Your unconscious mind helps you to make your thoughts a reality, so if you think, 'I'm fat', for example, then your unconscious mind will do everything it can to help you to be fat. You therefore need to make sure your thoughts reflect what you want.

Top Tip

Unsure about whether you have toxic thoughts? Remember that your body and life are a perfect reflection of your inner thoughts. So if you want to get an insight into the inner workings of your mind, simply look at your body and your life for clues.

Detox Your Thoughts
(time: 10 minutes)

Your conclusions about yourself impact every aspect of your body and life. In your journal, write down the conclusions you have come to about your body, your personality, your skills and abilities, relationships, money, career, health, and so on. To help you, complete the following sentences in your journal:

① I always get …
② I never feel …
③ I'm too …
④ II'll never …
⑤ It's hard to …
⑥ My body …

Examples of toxic conclusions are: 'I always eat food for comfort when I'm stressed' or 'I'm too old to start my own business'. Now write down what comes to mind when you think about the following:

① Family and friends
② Love and intimacy
③ Career and work
④ Money and wealth
⑤ Other

If there were some toxic conclusions in your lists you can now come to new ones. Conclusions have emotions attached to them, so to clear a toxic conclusion all you need to do is clear the emotion attached to it. Use the Mind Booster below to help you.

Optional mind booster
Coming to New Conclusions
(time: 2–3 minutes for each conclusion)

Let go of the old, out-of-date conclusions and they will transform back into passing thoughts that have little or no impact on your body or life. Think about the toxic conclusion you wish to cleanse, then:

① Relax your upper abdominal area (known as your solar plexus) just below your chest bone. Breathe deeply.

② Ask yourself what you now know that if you had known in the past, you would *never* have come to the old conclusion in the first place. You may find that the emotion associated with the conclusion disappears.

③ Ask yourself what you have been pretending *not* to know in order to keep the old conclusion going in your mind.

④ Finally, ask yourself what you need to acknowledge to be certain that the old conclusion has now served its purpose and is gone.

⑤ What would you prefer to believe instead of the old conclusion? Say the new conclusion three times to embed it into your unconscious mind. For example, if you want to lose weight, say 'I find it easy to stay in amazing shape', and create a picture in your mind's eye of how you would look if it were already the case. This will give your unconscious mind clear orders to follow.

Say your new conclusions frequently during your Life Detox – and beyond if necessary.

Your detox results
Look at the Life Detox goals and theme that you wrote down on Day 1 (page 85) and make sure you are taking steps to help yourself achieve them.

Goodnight journal questions
Answer the following questions in your journal:

① What was the best part of my day? (Take a moment to feel gratitude.)

② What have I done today to clear physical and emotional toxins from my body and life?

③ Why should I continue my Life Detox journey tomorrow?

dayfour tuesday

You need healthy blood to deliver life-giving oxygen to your body. Today works on purifying your blood and helps your lymphatic system operate well, too. We will also work through powerful ways to clear emotional toxins and feel more calm, confident and content.

Life Detox daily schedule

Upon rising 2 slices of lemon or lime in hot water

Morning mind detoxer Power-up Process (page 82)

Daily body exercise Yoga workout or skipping/rebounding (page 74)

Jump-out-of-bed juice Beetroot Blood Purifier, or fruit

Mid-morning raw-power snack Delicious Dip

Liver-loving lunch Greek Salad (page 135), plus choose one of the following options: 4 oatcakes, 4 rice cakes or 2 slices of rye bread (or other non-wheat bread)

Afternoon pick-me-up Mug of Life Detox Broth (page 127), or sachet of miso soup

Daytime mind detoxer Remove one to three items from your Toxic To-do List

Detox two-course dinner First course: Detox Salad (page 130); main course: Spanish-style Chickpeas with Wilted Spinach (page 136)

Optional body booster Dry skin brushing and massage

Evening mind detoxer Toxic Emotions Go!

Optional mind booster Use 3-C Vision to Feel Calm, Confident and Content

Just before bed Goodnight questions

For the body: Let Life Flow

Body detox daily update

For life to flow freely we depend on healthy blood to deliver oxygen to the rest of our body. We also depend on the lymphatic system, a network of glands and tubes that act as the cell's collection system, transporting waste to the other organs of elimination. Toxins can accumulate in these rivers of life and cause stagnation and imbalance throughout the rest of the body. Blood requires good nutrition – exactly what you will get by following our nutrition guidelines. The effects of detox on blood pressure and cholesterol can be quite amazing.

Are you familiar with your lymph glands? Perhaps you have felt the lymph nodes around the neck area. In a normal, healthy state they are about the size of almonds but they can become swollen and painful when you have been fighting an infection or when they are clogged up with excess toxins. Now is the time to give your lymph glands a helping hand. Today's body booster will improve the removal of waste materials between your organs and tissues, drain off excess fluids from the hips and thighs and relieve any residual water retention.

Today's juice: Beetroot Blood Purifier

Put 2 raw beetroots (peeled), 5 strawberries (stalks removed), 1 celery stick, ½ pineapple (peeled) and 2 apples through the juicer.

Fast facts about Beetroot Blood Purifier
Beetroots are a well-known blood tonic and have been used for centuries for this purpose alone. They are also now known for their powerful effect in helping to reduce bad LDL (low-density lipoprotein) cholesterol. The addition of flavoursome strawberries adds a mega dose of vitamin C – just five strawberries can give you your recommended daily allowance. Strawberries also contain the lesser-known vitamin K, necessary for effective blood clotting. Celery boosts the electrolyte balance of the body with a dose of organic sodium. These powerful ingredients blend perfectly with the juicy sweetness of nutritious pineapple.

Add one teaspoon of psyllium husks stirred quickly into the smoothie and follow with one 225ml (8fl oz) glass of water.

Delicious Dip

For your mid-morning raw-power snack, choose a handful of vegetable sticks or a piece of fruit of your choice and dip into 1–2 tbsp Raw Hummus or Guacamole (page 125).

Fluids and added extras

Remember to drink plenty of fluids and include your added extras as you did on Day 1 (page 79).

Body exercise

Include your minimum 15-minute yoga, skipping or rebounding workout (or your existing exercise programme) as described in Chapter 9 (page 74).

Optional body booster: dry skin brushing and massage

Dry skin brushing is easy for anyone to do at home.

Step 1 Dry skin brushing (time: 4–5 minutes)

Dry skin brushing is one of the most powerful ways to cleanse and exfoliate the skin and assist the job of the kidneys. It removes dead skin cells, clears the pores and stimulates the production of sebum – all of which help to improve the tone and texture of your skin. It also helps to cleanse the lymphatic system and increases blood circulation to the underlying organs and tissues in the body. Plus, it helps to break down cellulite. (Skin brushes are available from good chemists and natural suppliers; see Suppliers and Further Resources. Brushes must have bristles of vegetable origin, not nylon.)

Brush the skin *before* a bath or shower. Using a special skin brush, use clean sweeps in long, stroking movements, and always towards the heart. The strokes should feel firm and your skin will tingle afterwards. Try to cover the whole body (except the face).

Step 2 Massage

A professional massage will generally take 1 hour. However, if you are giving yourself a self-massage, aim for 20 minutes. If massaging at home, use comfortably warm organic massage oil.

Dip your fingertips into the warm oil and apply it lightly to the entire body. Wait for 4–5 minutes to let some of the oil be absorbed into your skin, then massage the entire body, applying even pressure with the whole hand. Apply light pressure on sensitive areas such as the abdomen. Use more oil and spend more time where nerve endings are concentrated, such as the soles of the feet, palms of the hands and along the base of the fingernails. Try to use circular motions over rounded areas and straight strokes on straight areas such as your arms and legs.

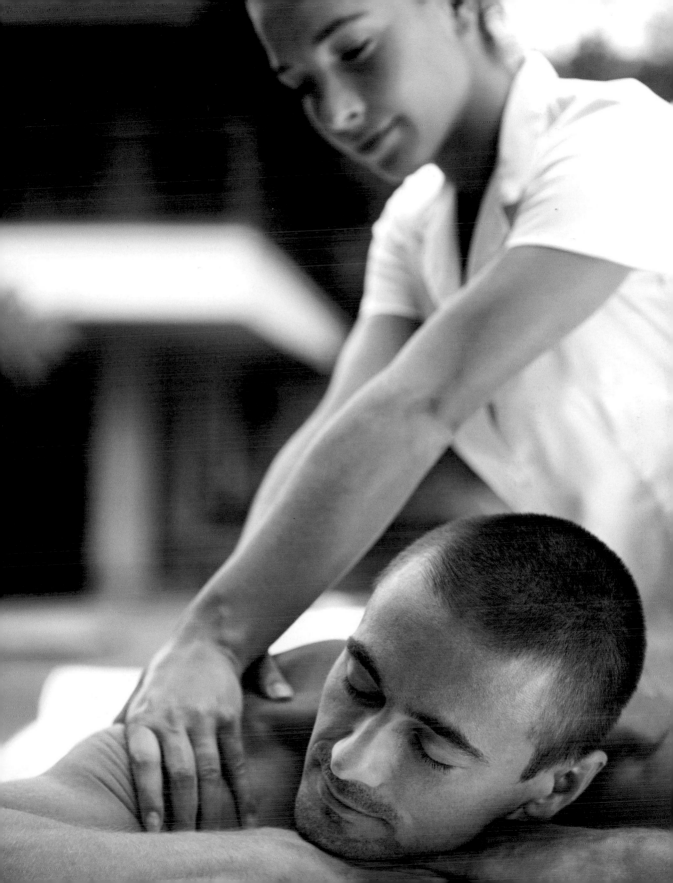

For the mind: Toxic Emotions Go!

Mind detox daily update

Today's the day to begin clearing out your toxic emotions. You may have noticed yourself feeling a bit 'emotional' during your detox. As you clear physical toxins it is normal to have emotional toxins come to the surface to clear, too. See our Evening Mind Detoxer.

Morning mind detoxer

Practise the Power-up Process from Day 1 when you first rise (page 82).

Daytime mind detoxer

Look at your Toxic To-do List from Day 1 (page 82) and deal with between one and three items so that they can be removed from the list.

Top Tips for dealing with toxic emotions

1. *If you're feeling angry*

Keep in mind that you cannot feel anger while you feel compassion. If a person is troubling you, rise above the way that you are presently seeing the problem and view the person or event from a different, more sympathetic and understanding perspective. Getting angry is the equivalent of drinking poison and expecting someone else to fall over and die! Your health is more important than any irritation or dispute.

2. *If you're feeling sad*

Remember your mind and body influence each other. To let go of sadness, think about the possible hidden benefits in difficult situations, because sadness cannot exist when you are thinking optimistic thoughts. You can also deal with sad feelings by making subtle changes to your body. Sit or stand with your spine erect, put your shoulders back, stick your chest out and up, breathe deeply and smile as you use 3-C Vision (explained on page 112). You'll be amazed at how much better you feel.

3. *If you're feeling fear*

You have a huge amount of life experience, knowledge, wisdom and other inbuilt resources that help to keep you safe and perform well. If you find yourself feeling fear, then use the energy generated by it to help you to focus your attention and enhance your performance. Remember, fear can only exist when you forget how amazingly resourceful you actually are.

4. *If you're feeling guilty*

If you are hard on yourself for your perceived failures by feeling guilty, then you can cause yourself unnecessary pain. Remember that you are perfect as you are (see See the Miracle in the Mirror, page 151), and you are always doing the best you can. It is completely natural to make mistakes once in a while. Rather than dwell on feeling guilty, focus on the lessons you can learn and do your best not make the same mistake again.

Evening mind detoxer

Emotions only become a problem if you don't let yourself feel them. So let your feelings flow! Clearing toxic emotions often requires you to think differently about those things that you have had problems with. Use today's exercises and detox booster to help you choose.

Toxic Emotions Go! (time: 2 minutes)

Follow these steps if you are feeling any toxic emotions:

① Relax your upper abdominal area; it can become tense through the build-up of unresolved toxic emotions. Breathe deeply by expanding your belly and letting your diaphragm drop. It will help the emotions to flow through your body.

② Acknowledge and accept your emotions' existence. If you don't, there is the possibility they could get stuck again. Accept the feelings as energy, and experience them without having to change them in any way.

③ Tell your unconscious mind what emotions you want. For example, if you are feeling anxious and nervous, then say, 'I am calm, confident and content', as if this is already how you feel.

Immediate Release for Stubborn Toxic Emotions (time: 2 minutes)

If the toxic emotions remain, it could mean that your unconscious mind isn't convinced that letting go of them is the safest and healthiest thing for you to do right now. Use the following questions to clear them.

① What do you know now, that if you had known in the past, you would *never* have felt the negative emotion? For example, if you are feeling angry towards another person, then you may now be aware that you are only hurting yourself by making yourself angry and if you had been more compassionate towards the other person, you would never have become angry in the first place.

② What have you been pretending *not* to know in order to keep the negative emotion?

A slightly odd question I admit, however, you will be amazed at how quickly the negative emotion disappears. For example, if you are feeling guilty about something you may have been pretending not to know that you can learn from your perceived mistakes. Knowing this can help you to stop regretting the past and instead start planning for the best-possible future.

③ What do you need to learn in order to let the emotion go easily? For example, if you are feeling anxious about what another person may think of you, then you may need to acknowledge that you only want to surround yourself with people who love you for who you are.

Optional mind booster

Use 3-C Vision to Feel Calm, Confident and Content (time: instant results)

Using 3-C vision is perhaps the quickest, easiest and most effective way to feel calm, confident and content. It can work instantly and in any situation. You can practice 3-C Vision by doing the following:

① Pick a spot on a wall to look at it, preferably above eye level, so that as you look at it it feels as though your vision is bumping up against your eyebrows. Make sure your eyes are not so high that you cut off your field of vision.

② As you stare at the spot on the wall, effortlessly let your mind go loose and focus all of your attention on the spot. At this point you may find yourself wanting to take a deep breath in and out. Let yourself do so.

③ Notice that within a matter of a few moments, your vision will begin to spread out. You will begin to see more in the peripheral than in the central part of your vision. You will feel it natural to take another couple of deep breaths in and out.

④ Now, pay more attention to the peripheral part of your vision than to the central part of your vision. Notice colours, shadows, shapes, and so on.

⑤ Continue for as long as you can while noticing how it feels. You will find calm, confident and content feelings come to you.

Use this technique during your daily life whenever you want to reduce your stress and feel calm, confident or content.

> **Your detox results**
> Look at the Life Detox goals and theme that you wrote down on Day 1 (page 85) and make sure you are taking steps to help yourself achieve them.

Goodnight journal questions

Answer the following questions in your journal:

① What was the best part of my day? (Take a moment to feel gratitude.)

② What have I done today to clear physical and emotional toxins from my body and life?

③ Why should I continue my Life Detox journey tomorrow?

dayfivewednesday

Using your lungs to their full potential is essential for good health, so today you will re-learn how to breathe! You will also cleanse the aspects of your self-image that may be toxic to your health, wealth, relationships and happiness.

LifeDetox daily schedule

Upon rising 2 slices of lemon or lime in hot water

Morning mind detoxer Power-up Process (page 82)

Daily body exercise Yoga workout or skipping/rebounding (page 74)

Jump- out-of-bed smoothie Veggie Apple Magic, or fruit

Mid-morning raw-power snack Delicious Dip

Liver-loving lunch Leftover Spanish-style Chickpeas with Wilted Spinach from Day 4, plus one of the following options: 4 oatcakes, 4 rice cakes or 2 slices of rye bread (or other non-wheat bread)

Afternoon pick-me-up A small handful of nuts and seeds (page 126)

Daytime mind detoxer Remove one to three items from your Toxic To-do List

Detox three-course dinner First course: Mug of Life Detox Broth (page 127), or sachet of miso soup; main course: Quinoa and Roast Vegetable Medley (page 137); dessert: Banana Ice Cream (page 138)

Optional body booster Belly breathing and child's pose (yoga)

Evening mind detoxer Boost Your Self-image

Optional mind booster Fountain of Feelings

Just before bed Goodnight questions

For the body: Boost Your Breathing

Body detox daily update

Today is all about breathing. The vast majority of people do not breathe properly and this has a dramatic impact on the body. What you breathe in is also important. Before you start today's optional body booster of belly breathing, we give you some helpful tips on clearing the air in your home.

A healing crisis

You might have experienced a runny nose this week. As the detox process moves forward, the lungs and the sinuses often begin to clear. A runny nose can be mistaken as the beginnings of a cold, and you may believe that you are feeling worse rather than better. This is what is called a 'healing crisis', when the body uses all its channels of elimination in the process of healing. Reactions vary from brief and mild to more intense and prolonged. If you are experiencing mucus secretions, drink warm water with a few slices of ginger between meals throughout the day. Ginger has been used for centuries in medical traditions to help release excess mucus.

Today's juice: Veggie Apple Magic

Put 3 carrots (scrubbed), 1 small cucumber, 1 celery stick and 2 apples (cored) through the juicer.

Add one teaspoon of psyllium husks stirred quickly into the smoothie and follow with one 225ml (8fl oz) glass of water.

Fast facts about Veggie Apple Magic
This is the ultimate alkalising juice! Apples have long been associated with detoxing, because of their high levels of pectin, a soluble fibre that helps to remove toxic waste from the intestines. Along with cucumber, they are highly alkalising and hydrating, which helps the blood to control levels of toxins. Carrots add a flavoursome punch and boost the antioxidant intake, in particular beta-carotene, well known for improving eyesight. With the addition of celery, a potent diuretic, this juice can help restore the correct water balance in the body.

Delicious Dip

For your mid-morning raw-power snack, choose a handful of vegetable sticks (pepper, carrot, courgette, cucumber, celery), or a piece of fruit of your choice and dip into 1–2 tbsp Raw Hummus or Guacamole (page 125).

Fluids and added extras

Remember to drink plenty of fluids and include your added extras as you did on Day 1 (page 79).

Body exercise

Include your minimum 15-minute yoga, skipping or rebounding workout (or your existing exercise programme) as described in Chapter 9 (page 74).

○○○○○○○○○○○○○○○○○○○○○○○○
Freshen up the air you breathe
Think about beginning today to cut down on the amount of chemicals you use in the home:
1. Switch from bleach, disinfectant and detergent to more natural cleaning products (see Suppliers and Further Resources).
2. Cut down on the use of perfume (other than natural perfumes), body sprays and other perfumed body products and use natural alternatives (see Suppliers and Further Resources).
3. Increase the number of plants in your indoor environment, as they help to improve the quality of the air.
○○○○○○○○○○○○○○○○○○○○○○○○

Optional body booster

Let's get to work on your breathing. Have you ever watched a baby sleep? You will see it is the belly and not the chest that rises and falls with each inhalation and exhalation. When we are born we instinctively use belly breathing. It is a simple technique that increases the range of movement used by the diaphragm, thus allowing the lungs to take in more oxygen and to release carbon dioxide more effectively. The relaxation that comes from belly breathing also improves our immune system. This slower, gentler movement encourages us to relax and withdraw for a few precious moments. These short spells of relaxation time can bring immeasurable long-term benefit.

Exercise: belly breathing (time: 5 minutes)
The belly breathing technique requires you to take a full breath in through your nose, filling your belly completely, and out through your mouth. The out-breath is twice as long as the in-breath.
① Lie down comfortably on your back on your bed, or a carpeted floor, or on a yoga mat. Put your feet flat on the floor and your knees bent (pointing upwards). Tune into your natural breathing for a few minutes.
② Place your hands one on top of the other on your navel.
③ Take a deep breath in through your nose, filling your lungs completely. Then exhale slowly through your mouth.
④ When you have tuned into the gentle rhythm of belly breathing, continue for 5 minutes more. Then, gently roll over to one side, and slowly sit up. If you have low blood

pressure, you may need to turn onto the left side first before sitting up, to avoid dizziness. Push yourself up gently by turning onto your right side.
⑤ Once you have completed 5 minutes of belly breathing, relax for a further 2 minutes in the soothing yoga posture called 'child's pose'.

Exercise: child's pose (time: 2 minutes)
① Kneel down with your bottom against the backs of your heels.
② Exhale and bend forward, gently resting your forehead on the floor. Your knees are tucked into your chest.
③ Have your arms by your sides, with the palms facing up.
④ Relax and breathe into the pose.

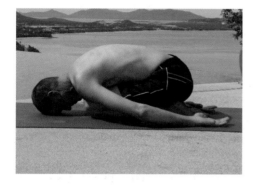

For the mind: Boost Your Self-image

Mind detox daily update
Today you are going to cleanse those aspects of your personal identity that may be toxic to your body and life. Because your identity shapes the choices you make, it is vital that it supports the body and life you want. See today's evening mind exercise to find out more.

Morning mind detoxer
Practise the Power-up Process from Day 1 when you first rise (page 82).

Daytime mind detoxer
Look at your Toxic To-do List from Day 1 (page 82) and deal with between one and three items so that they can be removed from the list.

Evening mind detoxer
You are what you think you are, and you will become what you think you will become. Your unconscious mind is designed to do what it's told. If you think about yourself as a passionate, confident, adventurous, creative and

motivated person, then over time your mind will help you to be that person. However, the same is also true if you see yourself as a dull, timid, unhealthy failure. If you suffer from a poor self-image, then use today's exercise and detox booster to improve it.

Boost Your Self-image (time: 5 minutes)
You are going to write down a positive statement that will help you to improve your self-image. Choose some aspirational words to say about yourself that could go into this statement. For example, 'I am an inspiring leader who steps up and makes a difference!' You might find the following lists useful:

Words to describe yourself:
Incredible, passionate, beautiful, powerful, dynamic, joyful, generous, energetic, gorgeous, strong, decisive, legendary, unstoppable, curious, fabulous, special, sexy, loving, funny, interesting, extraordinary, giving, adventurous, creative, energised, stunning, resourceful, inspiring, exotic, wealthy, happy, honest, kind, superb, helpful, wise.

What you are or would like to be:
Leader, winner, helper, listener, teacher, coach, guide, lover, friend, role model, artist, achiever, entertainer, trainer, soul mate, champion, team player, mother, father, son, daughter, brother, sister, millionaire, icon, philosopher, hero, beautiful, spirit, public speaker.

Your qualities: Inspires others, steps up, makes a difference, rocks, motivates others, loves unconditionally, accepts others, gets results, sets new standards, shines, listens, loves life, laughs, succeeds.

Say your self-image statement every day as if you already believe it is true. Write it down; you may need to refer to it until it is memorised.

Today's Top Tip:
Always base your self-image upon your intentions rather than your mistakes. This is liberating because, instead of identifying yourself with the low points in your life, you focus on your highest intentions, which are always positive and loving.

Optional mind booster
Fountain of Feelings (time: 3 minutes)
Boost your new self-image by associating it with positive feelings.

Doing this will help you to believe your positive statement about yourself even quicker.
① Decide how you want to feel (confident, contented, peaceful, and so on). Relax your body and take a couple of deep breaths.

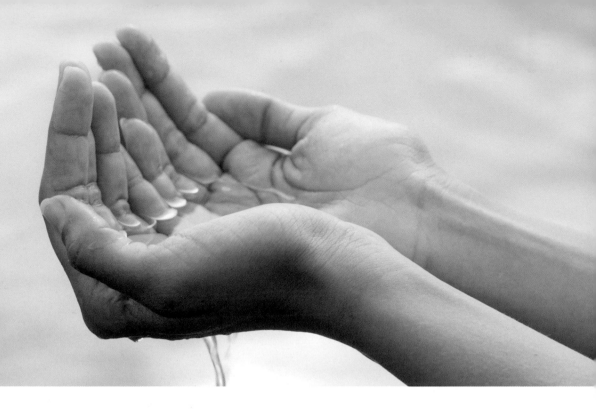

② If the feeling you want had a colour, what would it be? Imagine a coloured fountain of that feeling flowing in front of you. Make the colour even more vibrant.

③ If the feeling had a sound, what would the sound be? Listen to it now.

④ If the feeling had a texture, how would it feel? Cup your hands in front of you and place them under the abundant flow of the fountain of feeling.

⑤ Imagine drinking the feeling from your cupped hands. See the colour, hear the sounds and feel the feeling as it enters your mouth and becomes absorbed into your body. Keep drinking until you know you are filled up.

⑥ Now imagine your fountain of feeling creating a fine mist. The mist surrounds your entire body. Breathe it in and let it be absorbed and circulate around your entire body. Feel it cleansing, purifying and energising. Take three more deep breaths.

⑦ End by saying three times each: 'It is done', then 'I am full', and finally, 'Thank you'.

Goodnight journal questions
Answer the following questions in your journal:

① What was the best part of my day? (Take a moment to feel gratitude.)

② What have I done today to clear physical and emotional toxins from my body and life?

③ Why should I continue my Life Detox journey tomorrow?

day**six**thursday

Your skin is your body's largest organ of elimination. Today focuses on ways to help it look and feel great. You will also learn how to reduce the negative effects of stress on your body and mind.

LifeDetox daily schedule

Upon rising 2 slices of lemon or lime in hot water

Morning mind detoxer Power-up Process (page 82)

Daily body exercise Yoga workout or skipping/rebounding (page 74)

Jump-out-of-bed smoothie Popeye's Punch, or fruit

Mid-morning raw-power snack Delicious Dip

Two-course liver-loving lunch Leftover Quinoa and Roast Vegetable Medley from Day 5, plus one of the following options: 4 oatcakes, 4 rice cakes or 2 slices of rye bread (or other non-wheat bread)

Afternoon pick-me-up Mug of Life Detox Broth (page 127), or sachet of miso soup

Daytime mind detoxer Remove one to three items from your Toxic To-do List

Detox two-course dinner First course: Detox Salad (page 130); main course: Spicy Scrambled Eggs with Herb Salsa (page 138) and 2 rough oatcakes

Optional body booster Sauna and home-made skin care

Evening mind detoxer Sort out the Stress

Optional mind booster Power of Appreciation

Just before bed Goodnight questions

For the body: Shape up the Skin

Body detox daily update

We often think of skin in an aesthetic way only: how good it looks, how young it looks – but remember: it is also a major organ of elimination. One of the most common side-effects of detoxing is an outbreak on the skin. Sometimes that means a pimple, at other times it could be a rash or even a temporary flare-up of eczema. If you have experienced some kind of skin reaction then you should be pleased with yourself, because it means that your largest living organ, your skin, is working well. The skin is one of our most responsive organs and is an honest reflection of the life we lead. When we detox, toxins start to move from deeper areas of the body to the more superficial organs, including the skin.

There is sometimes a brief reaction as your body cleanses – think of it as the toxins bidding you a fond farewell. This is not to say that chronic skin problems are a good sign; on the contrary, they often reflect deeper problems. Lacklustre or dull skin indicates deficiencies in essential vitamins and minerals; pale skin can be a sign of low iron or anaemia; dry skin can indicate a deficiency in essential oils; and skin problems such as acne or eczema are often linked to a weak digestion – which can be inherited as well as created through lifestyle. No matter what your skin type, try to find some extra time today to pamper yourself and shape up your skin, naturally.

Using a sauna

If you have access to a sauna, preferably of the infrared variety, then please try to book yourself in for a session. Sweating is an important elimination route for the body, and a sauna is a great way to flush out large amounts of toxins. To ensure you are comfortable, avoid eating your main meal for two hours before a sauna session and make sure you drink a minimum of 225ml (8fl oz) of water before entering. Follow the sauna's guidelines on removing jewellery and the length of time permitted, as not all saunas are the same.

To enhance the effects, visualise absorbing the heat and energy. Deep, slow breathing and maintaining good posture are also helpful. Please note, if you are a man trying for a baby then do not use saunas, as high temperatures can affect the quantity and quality of your sperm.

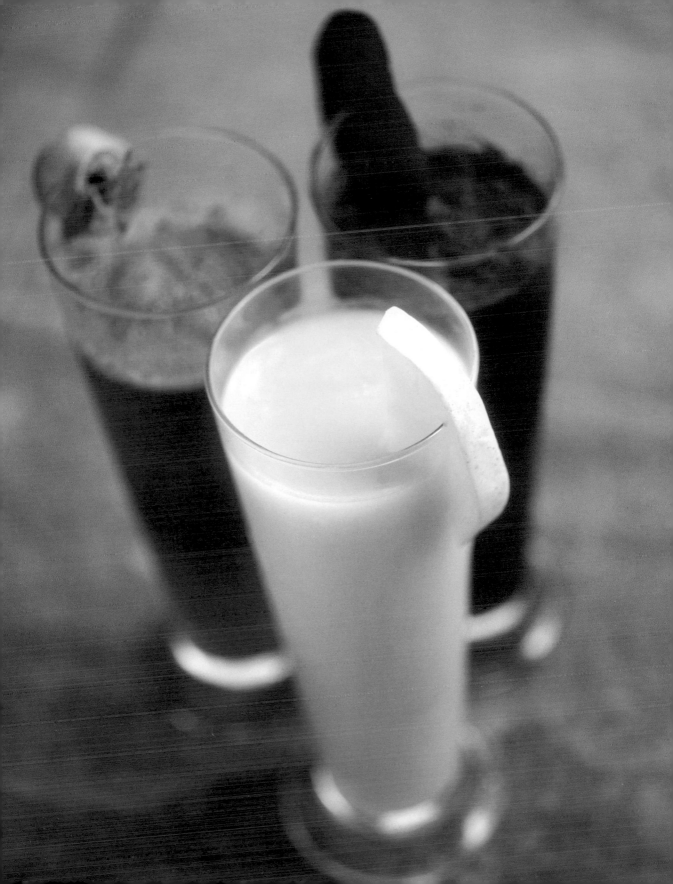

Today's smoothie: Popeye's Punch

Blend together 1 handful of baby spinach, 1 small cucumber, ½ pineapple (peeled), 2 apples (cored), 1 lemon (peeled) ½ avocado.

Add one teaspoon of psyllium husks stirred quickly into the smoothie and follow with one 225ml (8fl oz) glass of water.

Fast facts about Popeye's Punch
The carton character Popeye made spinach famous, thanks to its strength-giving iron content. The addition of lemon in this smoothie helps to make the iron more easily absorbed. The green leaves are given their colour by chlorophyll, which acts as a powerful cleanser. Avocados are rich in beautifying vitamin E – perfect for skin suppleness – and are reputed to be a sexual tonic! There is no need to worry about the fat content, as avocados contain healthy monosaturated fat, which also helps to keep blood sugar stable, giving you energy throughout the morning. This smoothie is sweetened by the pineapple and apple, both helpful for detoxification.

Delicious Dip

For your mid-morning raw-power snack, choose a handful of vegetable sticks (pepper, carrot, courgette, cucumber, celery), or a piece of fruit of your choice and dip into 1–2 tbsp Raw Hummus or Guacamole (page 125).

Fluids and added extras

Remember to drink plenty of fluids and include your added extras as you did on Day 1 (page 78).

Body exercise

Include your minimum 15-minute yoga, skipping or rebounding workout (or your existing exercise programme) as described in Chapter 9 (page 74).

Optional body booster: sauna and home-made skin care

Here's how to give your skin a boost from the inside and outside:
Step 1 Repeat dry skin brushing (see Day 4, page 100).
Step 2 Go for a sauna if possible.
Step 3 Treat yourself to some home-made skin care. You might like to make our lovely Oats and Citrus Deep Cleanser that can be used on your body or face (suitable for a combination/dry skin).

Oats and Citrus Deep Cleanser

This is an exfoliating cleanser to be used twice a week and is suitable for the face and body. You can add a few drops of your chosen essential oil to the mixture, if you like.
100g (3½oz) oats
grated rind of 1 lemon

grated rind of 1 orange

½ tsp dried thyme

① Put all the ingredients in a food processor and process to a powder, or use a pestle and mortar. Put the mixture in a fine muslin bag or a coffee filter until the lemon rind is totally dry, then store in an airtight container.

② To use, just add water to a teaspoonful of the powder in the palm of your hand and mix to form a paste. Apply by patting onto the skin. Dampen your hands to work it in – press, don't rub, then rinse it off with lukewarm water. The dried preparation will last until the expiry date of the oats you have used.

For the mind: Sort out the Stress

Mind detox daily update

Prolonged stress harms your body and can lead you to perform less well, compared to when you are calm, relaxed and able to think clearly and creatively. Sorting out the stress is about stepping off the treadmill of 'having to get things done', and instead making your health and well-being your number-one priority. Our evening mind detoxer explains how to reduce your stress.

Morning mind detoxer

Practise the Power-up Process from Day 1 when you first rise (page 82).

Daytime mind detoxer

Look at your Toxic To-do List from Day 1 (page 91) and deal with between one and three items so that they can be removed from the list.

Evening mind detoxer

Stress cannot exist if we simply accept a situation. Say you're running late for an appointment. The mental and emotional stress of your lateness causes biochemical changes in your body. However, it's not being late that causes these changes. It's your resistance to being late that does.

Sort out the Stress (time: 5 minutes)

List the things in your life that are currently causing you stress. Use the following headings as a guide:

☺ Family and friends

☺ Life partner

☺ Past relationships

☺ Other relationships

☺ Career and work

☺ Health and vitality

☺ Money and wealth

☺ Living environment

As you think about the things on your list, go through them one-by-one and notice how you feel when you stop resisting the current situation and totally accept it.

Stop Stressing Now (time: 5 minutes)

If any stressful situation is hard to accept, then answering the following questions can help you to change how you're thinking about it:

① What's been stopping you from being stress-free? Have you stopped yourself from relaxing because you fear not being good enough, not being loved, not getting what you think you want or losing what you've got?

② How have you benefited from being stressed? What is it that you enjoy doing, which you won't be able to do when the stress disappears?

③ What do you need to learn in order to let go of the stress now? Now that you've learned it, it's OK for the stress to go. If not, what else do you need to acknowledge?

④ Why should you free yourself from the stress now? How will you benefit by letting go of it now? How will your relationships improve, your health and your wealth? How will your life become more fulfilling? Take a moment to enjoy how it feels to know you are free now.

Doing the above exercise using today's booster improves the results.

Optional mind booster

Power of Appreciation (time: 5 minutes)

A study published in 1995 showed that appreciative thoughts put less stress on the body compared with angry thoughts. Appreciative thoughts caused smooth and regular heart rhythms whereas thoughts of anger and frustration caused uneven and irregular heart rhythms. This highlights how important it is to approach life with a positive and grateful attitude.

For each of the areas of your life that you have been getting stressed about (see list on page 115), write in your journal all the things you are grateful for instead. This will help you appreciate what's right instead of focusing on what's wrong.

Your detox results

Look at the Life Detox goals and theme that you wrote down on Day 1 (page 85) and make sure you are taking steps to help yourself achieve them.

Goodnight journal questions

Answer these in your journal:

① What was the best part of my day? (Take a moment to feel gratitude.)

② What have I done today to clear physical and emotional toxins from my body and life?

③ Why should I continue my Life Detox journey tomorrow?

daysevenfriday

Today's the day for giving your body a well-deserved treat, and you will learn how to energise your mind in a special way so that it continues to help you create the body and life you want.

LifeDetox daily schedule

Upon rising 2 slices of lemon or lime in hot water

Morning mind detoxer Power-up Process (page 82)

Daily body exercise Yoga workout or skipping/rebounding (page 74)

Jump-out-of-bed juice Detox Zinger, or fruit

Mid-morning raw-power snack Delicious Dip

Liver-loving lunch Moroccan Avocado Salad (page 139), plus one of the following options: 4 oatcakes, 4 rice cakes or 2 slices of rye bread (or other non-wheat bread)

Afternoon pick-me-up A small handful of nuts and seeds (page 126)

Daytime mind detoxer Remove one to three items from your Toxic To-do List

Detox two-course dinner Main course: Sweet Potato Green Curry with Fish or Tofu (page 140); dessert: Banana Berry Bake (page 141)

Optional body booster Home hydrotherapy and treat yourself!

Evening mind detoxer Energise Your Mind

Optional mind booster Getting Your Goals

Just before bed Goodnight questions

For the body: Energise Your Body

Body detox daily update

Congratulations – you have made it to Day 7! Not only can you feel good in yourself, but also today is a great time to treat your body for all its hard work. Perhaps in the past you would have opted for some indulgent food or wine, but this is not a good idea straight after detox. So this time it is all about giving your body a real treat, inside and out. For those of you who have been aiming for weight loss, wait until tomorrow morning before standing on the scales again.

Moving on to the next stage

Your 7-day detox finishes today so you should now think about whether you would like to take the ultimate weight-loss boost with our 24-hour turbo-detox day tomorrow (see page 145). Although it is a very powerful step, it is easier than it sounds – but it does require slowing down other demands, so try to make sure you don't plan much else in your diary.

Even if you are ready to finish your detox today, it is our not-so-secret desire that you will have fallen in love with your new way of eating and decide to make it a way of life. At the very least, the first few days after a detox are especially important because your body needs to be eased out of detox gently. Celebrating should not involve alcohol for a few days at least – we have had several phone calls from detox clients who have decided to 'celebrate' the end of a detox with a glass of wine and have promptly thrown up! This is because your body is in healing mode and can reject toxic substances with greater force.

Today's juice: Detox Zinger

Put 8 carrots (scrubbed), 2 apples (cored) and a small piece of fresh root ginger (peeled) through the juicer.

Add one teaspoon of psyllium husks stirred quickly into the juice and follow with one 225ml (8fl oz) glass of water.

Fast facts about today's juice: Detox Zinger
End your detox week on a high with the refreshing taste of this zinger. The ginger is not only good for digestion but also boosts circulation and can even help relieve allergies. Carrots, as well as the apples, contain good levels of pectin, a special fibre that has cholesterol-lowering properties. They are also a great source of folic acid and magnesium.

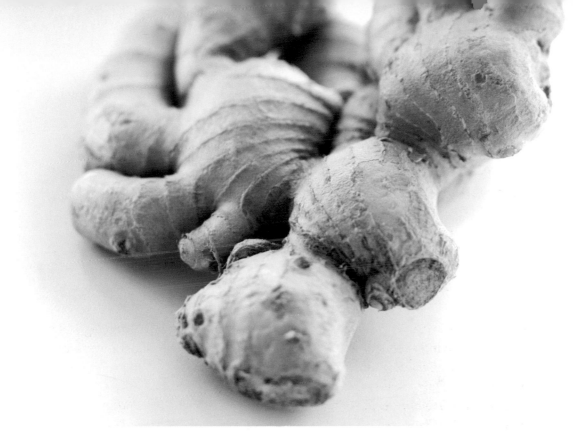

Delicious Dip

For your mid-morning raw-power snack, choose a handful of vegetable sticks (pepper, carrot, courgette, cucumber, celery), or a piece of fruit of your choice and dip into 1–2 tbsp Raw Hummus or Guacamole (page 125).

Fluids and added extras

Remember to drink plenty of fluids and include your added extras as you did on Day 1 (pages 79–85).

Body exercise

Include your minimum 15-minute yoga, skipping or rebounding workout (or your existing exercise programme) as described in Chapter 10 (page 74).

Optional body booster: treat yourself!

If you thought you would be winding down by now, think again. We want you to feel energetic and full of vitality! Today's booster is the simplest yet, but the first part – hydrotherapy – requires some mental toughness. Don't worry; you get to treat yourself once the shower is over!

Home hydrotherapy

For home hydrotherapy all you need to do is take a cold shower for at least 15 seconds, but preferably for 1 minute. Although this may sound like torture rather than a pleasure, cold showers are extremely effective at boosting circulation. If you have ever plunged into a cold pool you will know that it is an extremely invigorating experience.

And now for the treat

For those of you that have associated a 'treat' with sweet foods or a glass of wine then this is a real learning curve for you. Those are not treats as far as your body is concerned. So, this treat has to be *truly* for your body. Here are a few suggestions:

☺ Book in for a massage.

☺ Go for a natural facial.

☺ Have another Epsom salts bath, but this time make sure it is by candlelight.

☺ Go to a yoga class.

☺ Go for a sauna.

☺ Go for a walk in an area of natural beauty.

☺ Book in for a horse-riding lesson.

☺ Go for an exhilarating cycle around a park or on a woodland route.

☺ Have a romantic night in (or book a hotel) with your partner – use your imagination.

☺ Go for a colonic – not everyone's idea of a treat, but you feel great afterwards!

You're sure to have other ideas – be inventive and make it personal to you.

For the mind: Energise Your Mind

Mind detox daily update

Today you are going to get clear about your goals and discover how to focus on them in a special way so that you can more easily achieve them. See today's evening mind detoxer.

Morning mind detoxer

Practise the Power-up Process from Day 1 when you first rise (page 82).

Daytime mind detoxer

Look at your Toxic To-do List from Day 1 (page 82) and deal with between one and three items so that they can be removed from the list.

Evening mind detoxer

Think of your conscious mind as the goal setter and your unconscious mind as the goal getter. You need to make sure your unconscious mind is making you aware of all the things you need to get your goals. You can become like a magnet to your goals and aspirations, simply by energising your mind.

Energise Your Mind (time: 10–25 minutes)
In your journal, write your age now and what your age will be in five years' time. Following the headings opposite, think about your true desires. How would these aspects of your life be in five years' time? Now write the story of your future in the present tense, as if you have already achieved all the goals you want. For example, 'My body is …; my life partner is …; I work as …; my home is …; I spend my time …', and so on. Write as much detail as possible.

Body (including shape, size, skin, energy, and general health)

Relationships (including family, friends, colleagues, life partner etc)

Career and work (including type of work, hours, values fulfilled, development, and so on)

Money and wealth (including how much you want, savings, investments, to be debt-free, etc)

Living environment (including where and with whom, etc)

Hobbies and interests (including where you travel, social activities and what you do with your spare time)

Optional mind booster

Getting Your Goals (time: 5 minutes)

Your unconscious mind filters your reality and passes a vastly edited version of life events up to your conscious awareness. You need to make sure you notice all the things that will help you to accomplish your goals. This booster will activate your unconscious mind.

① What is the very last thing that has to happen for you to know you've achieved your goal? Imagine what you will see, hear, feel, smell and taste when you've got it. For example, if you want a new house, imagine waking up in the new house a couple of weeks after you've moved in. By that point you will know for sure that you have achieved your goal.

② Let yourself tune into and fully feel what it will be like to have accomplished your goal; spend anything from 1 to 5 minutes doing this.

③ In your mind's eye, shrink the image of yourself getting your goal down to the size of a postcard. Visualise gently placing the image of what you want in the palm of your hand. Appreciate it now as if you've already attracted it into your life.

④ Take four very deep breaths, breathing each of them into your goal. With each breath, see your goal become more energised and full of life force.

⑤ Now imagine your goal flying into your future to manifest at a time that is most perfect for you, but do not give it a specific date (as this may delay it!).

Repeat this detox booster a couple of times a week (if required) until you have your goal.

Your detox results
Look at the Life Detox goals and theme that you wrote down on Day 1 (page 93) and make sure you have achieved them. If not, you may choose to complete them over the next few days.

Goodnight journal questions

Answer the following questions in your journal:

① What was the best part of my detox week? (Take a moment to feel gratitude.)

② What have I done this week to clear physical and emotional toxins from my body and life?

③ Do I want to continue my Life Detox journey tomorrow with a turbo-detox day? (See page 145 to find out how.)

chapter eleven

Life Detox 7-Day Programme Recipes

To help your Life Detox 7-Day Programme run smoothly, all your recipes are included here. The emphasis on our recipes has been to use fresh, organic ingredients and as many raw foods as possible, so you may be surprised to see that our hummus, for example, is actually a raw version using soaked cashew nuts instead of chickpeas. If you can't manage to prepare all the recipes, try to buy organic for as many of your meals as possible; for example, organic soup or organic ready-made hummus.

As well as your main meals and snacks, remember that you have a daily allowance of the following:

2 tbsp olive oil (for cooking or for a salad dressing)
1 tsp butter (for spreading)
2 tbsp linseed (flax) oil (for a salad dressing or in smoothies)

Your week's recipes at a glance

Day 1 Tomato and Bean Soup, Detox Salad, Chilli con Veggie
Day 2 Leftover Chilli con Veggie, leftover Tomato and Bean Soup, Warm Butternut and Goat's Cheese Salad, Stewed Apples with Blueberries or Compote
Day 3 Butternut and Carrot Soup, leftover Stewed Apples with Blueberries or Compote, Baked Fish with Rosemary Roasted Veggies
Day 4 Greek Salad, Detox Salad, Spanish-style Chickpeas with Wilted Spinach
Day 5 Leftover Spanish-style Chickpeas with Wilted Spinach, Quinoa and Roast Vegetable Medley, Banana Ice Cream
Day 6 Leftover Quinoa and Roast Vegetable Medley, Detox Salad, Spicy Scrambled Eggs with Herb Salsa
Day 7 Moroccan Avocado Salad, Sweet Potato Green Curry with Fish or Tofu, Banana Berry Bake

Every day

You begin each day with a fresh juice or smoothie. The ingredients are listed in your daily programme.

You will need a juicer and a blender to make the delicious juices and smoothies for the 7-day programme (see Suppliers and Further Resources). When juicing, there is no need to peel fruits such as apples and carrots, although they need to be washed first. Apples need to be cored. The whole fruit is usually added to the juice extractor. Drink the juice as soon as you have made it. When making a smoothie, chop the fruit into chunks before adding to the blender with the liquid.

Each day your mid-morning snack is a raw-power snack of vegetables and dip to keep you going until lunchtime. Making dips is quick and easy and they are cheaper to make than to buy. Making your own also cuts down on the number of plastic containers you have in your shopping trolley. However, if you do not have time to make the dips, please try to buy ones made with organic ingredients.

Raw-power Snack

Chop up any vegetable that can be eaten raw into crudité-size dipping pieces. Choose from pepper, carrot, courgette, cucumber, celery, cauliflower or broccoli.

Raw Hummus

This is a different take on hummus (more tasty, actually), and was designed by a world-class raw-food chef. It keeps the diet powerful all the way till lunchtime.

SERVES 2–3
100g (3 ½oz) cashew nuts, soaked overnight and drained
2 tsp lemon juice
5 tsp olive oil
1–2 garlic cloves
pinch of sea salt
pinch of ground cumin or cayenne pepper
chopped fresh parsley and ground paprika, to garnish

① In a food processor or blender, blend the cashew nuts, lemon, olive oil and garlic, with enough water to combine until smooth.
② Add the sea salt and cumin or cayenne pepper. Transfer to a serving bowl and garnish with parsley and paprika.

Guacamole

Avocados are rich in essential oils and taste great. Guacamole is easy to make and exceptionally tasty.

SERVES 2–3
½ avocado
juice of ¼ lemon
1 tsp finely chopped red onion
pinch of sea salt
1 tsp olive oil

① Cut the avocado into halves. Remove the stone and scoop out the flesh into a small bowl. Use a fork to mash the avocado.
② Stir in the lemon juice, onion, salt and olive oil. Cover the bowl and refrigerate for 1 hour before serving.

Afternoon pick-me-ups

During the afternoon a healthy snack of nuts and seeds or warming broth will keep you going when your energy needs a boost.

Nuts and seeds (unsalted)

Apart from containing valuable essential fatty acids, nuts and seeds are also high in the minerals zinc and selenium. These two minerals are key antioxidant minerals and are needed to activate a variety of detox processes. Nuts and seeds also contain essential fats and provide a good source of protein. Choose from brazil nuts, almonds, cashew nuts, hazelnuts, macadamia nuts, pecan nuts, pine nuts, pistachio nuts and walnuts. No peanuts. Unsalted seeds (such as sesame, pumpkin and sunflower) are good, too.

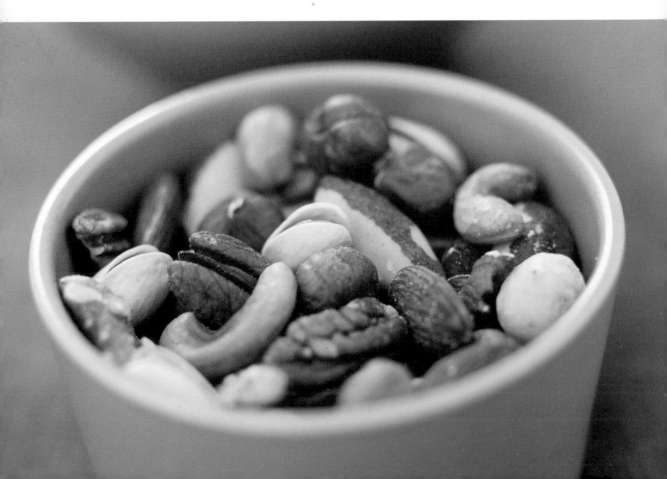

Life Detox Broth

This broth is the ultimate detox cocktail. Rich in minerals and vitamins, it helps to balance the pH of the body, promoting cleansing of all the body tissues, as well as balancing electrolytes. If you sweat often, from exercise or saunas, then increase your intake of the detox broth. You can vary the taste by adding any spice except salt – cayenne pepper is especially good for a detox. As an alternative to the broth, you can have miso soup for your afternoon pick-me-up. Miso, which is made from fermented soya beans, is full of nutrients and the healthy soup can be quickly made from a sachet.

MAKES ABOUT 2.8 LITRES (5 PINTS)
4 large potatoes, chopped
6 carrots, chopped
1 head of celery, including the leaves, chopped
1 small bunch of green vegetables, such as broccoli, kale
or green beans, chopped
1 apple, cored and chopped
1 bunch of chopped fresh herbs, such as parsley, oregano or coriander

① Fill your largest pan (preferably stainless steel) with 2.8 litres (5 pints) water. Put all the vegetables into the pan with the apple and half the herbs. Bring to the boil then simmer gently for a minimum of 1½ hours, or up to 3 hours for a more intense flavour. ② Remove from the heat and strain off all vegetables and fruit. Consume only the broth liquid and add the remaining herbs before serving. Store in the refrigerator for three days or freeze.

Life Detox Salad Dressing

This is a light and tasty salad dressing that is healthy as well as great for transforming any salad.

SERVES 1
1 tbsp olive oil
1–2 tbsp linseed (flax) oil
squeeze of fresh lemon juice
1 tbsp cider vinegar
freshly ground black pepper

Put all the ingredients in a screw-top jar and shake them together well.

Day 1

Chilli con Veggie

This is a lovely spicy mix and there will be enough for you to use for lunch tomorrow. Serve with the Detox Salad.

SERVES 2

200g (7oz) kidney beans, soaked overnight, drained and rinsed, or 400g (14oz) can kidney beans, drained and rinsed
1 tbsp olive oil
$^1/_4$–$^1/_2$ tsp chilli powder
$^1/_4$ tsp ground cumin
$^1/_4$ tsp ground turmeric
3 celery sticks, chopped
1 green or red pepper, chopped
2 carrots, chopped
2 tomatoes, chopped
4 tbsp tomato purée
squeeze of fresh lemon juice, to taste

① Place the soaked and rinsed dried kidney beans, if using, in a pan, cover with water and bring to the boil for 15 minutes. Simmer for a further 1–1$^1/_2$ hours, or until the beans are very tender. Drain and set aside.
② Heat the oil in a large pan and fry the spices for 1–2 minutes. Add the celery, pepper and carrots, and cook until soft.
③ Stir in the tomatoes and tomato purée, and cook for a further 10–15 minutes, stirring frequently. Add the beans and cook for a further 10 minutes. Serve with a squeeze of fresh lemon juice.

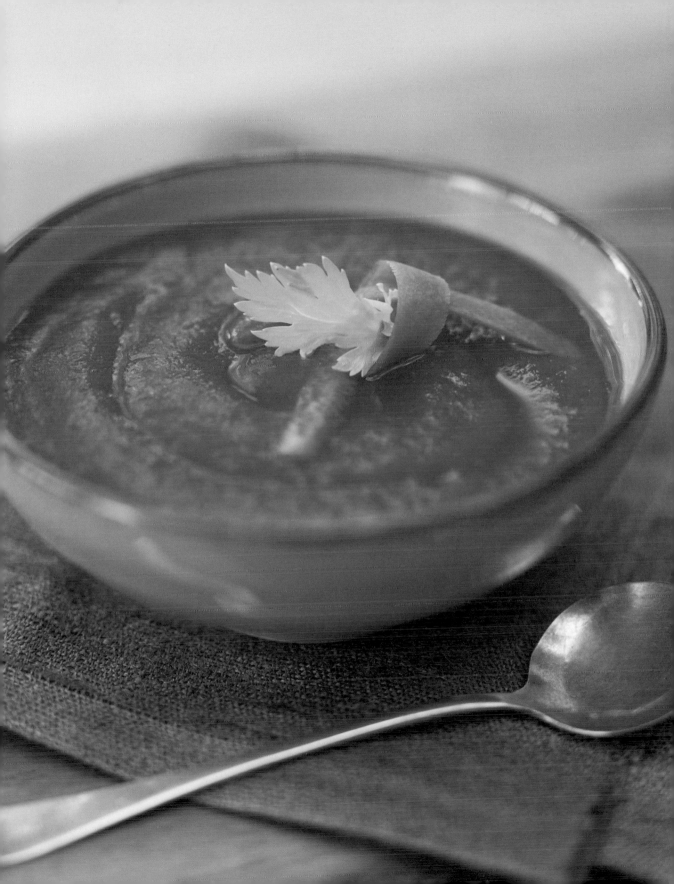

Detox Salad

Choose a variety of salad leaves to give you the best flavour when you make this fresh-tasting salad that tastes great with the Life Detox Salad Dressing (page 127).

SERVES 1
handful of seasonal salad leaves, torn
3 small tomatoes or 1 large tomato, sliced
1 small carrot, grated or julienned (cut into thin matchsticks)
¼ cucumber, diced, or a few radishes

Toss all the ingredients together. Serve drizzled with Life Detox Salad Dressing (page 127).

Variation

Add ½ celery stick, chopped, or use rocket or watercress instead of lettuce.

Tomato and Bean Soup

A tasty and filling bean soup that will be enough for lunch on Day 1 and as a first course on Day 2.

SERVES 2
1 large onion, chopped
1 tbsp olive oil
115g (4oz) butter beans, soaked overnight, drained and rinsed, or 200g (7oz) can, drained and rinsed
400g (14oz) can tomatoes or 700g (1lb 9oz) jar passata
1 bay leaf
1 litre (1¾ pints) vegetable stock (low-sodium variety or home-made)
freshly ground black pepper

① Fry the onion in the olive oil until soft but not browned. Add the butter beans, tomatoes or passata, and the bay leaf, and cook for 3 minutes more.
② Add the stock and bring to the boil. Simmer for 30 minutes for pre-cooked beans or 1–1½ hours for uncooked beans.
③ Remove the bay leaf and process the soup in a liquidiser or blender until smooth.

Variations

Add some carrots or celery, or spice it up with some deseeded and chopped chillies. The soup can also be served with crumbled goat's cheese.

Day 2

Warm Butternut and Goat's Cheese Salad

Our household is crazy about large salads; it feels like you have a large meal yet you feel light and energetic afterwards – perfect for the evenings. This one is particularly tasty. Feel free to experiment with some additional ingredients such as pine nuts or roasted tomatoes.

SERVES I

½ small butternut squash, flesh cut into 1cm (½in) cubes
200g (7oz) seasonal salad leaves, washed
150g (5½oz) baby spinach leaves, washed
1 carrot, grated
1 red onion, chopped finely
75g (3oz) sprouted mung beans (optional)
6 baby plum tomatoes or cherry tomatoes, or 3–5 sun-blush tomatoes
120g (4oz) goat's or sheep's cheese, cubed
Life Detox Salad Dressing (page 127), to serve

① Preheat the oven to 180°C/350°F/Gas 4. Place the butternut squash in a lightly oiled roasting pan and bake until soft, about 30 minutes.
② Combine all the remaining salad ingredients in a large salad bowl, keeping the squash warm in the oven until ready to serve.
③ Grill the goat's or sheep's cheese on a piece of baking parchment until lightly browned. Remove and add to the salad with the butternut squash. Drizzle over Life Detox Salad Dressing (page 135).

Stewed Apples with Blueberries

This was an absolute favourite in Amanda's family while she was growing up. There is enough here for two meals, so serve half the apples with your chosen topping for dessert today and save the other half for tomorrow's lunch.

SERVES 2

2 large cooking apples, peeled and chopped
¼ tsp powdered cinnamon (optional)
2 tbsp blueberries or 1 tbsp Compote (page 132), to serve

① Put the apples in a pan and add 3 tbsp water. Cook over a very gentle heat, adding cinnamon, if you like.

② Remove from the heat once soft. Serve with fresh blueberries or Compote.

Compote

Delicious hot or cold, on its own or used with stewed apples, this compote is made with mineral-rich dried fruit. Preparation starts the night before, as the fruit needs to soak overnight. It is best to make a batch and keep it for a few days in the refrigerator.

SERVES 2

3 dried apricots
3 dried apples
3 dried prunes
150ml (¼ pint) apple juice
1 cinnamon stick
3 cloves

① Put all the fruit in a bowl and pour over the apple juice and water to cover. Soak overnight.

② The next day, transfer the mixture to a pan, with the cinnamon stick and cloves. Add water to cover, if necessary, and bring the mixture to the boil. Simmer gently for 20-25 minutes. Remove the spices and serve.

Day 3

Butternut and Carrot Soup

A great low-calorie energy booster that is full of beta-carotene. It is simple and nourishing; ideal when you need to be warmed from the inside. The recipe serves 4 so you could freeze three portions to use during your pH-Principle Diet, or share it with others, as it makes an excellent lunch.

SERVES 4
1 onion, chopped
4 garlic cloves, chopped
1 tbsp olive oil
4 carrots: 1 grated and 3 sliced
1 celery stick, chopped
½ butternut squash, flesh roughly chopped
1.2 litres (2 pints) vegetable stock (low-sodium variety or home-made)
50ml (2fl oz) soya milk (optional)
freshly ground black pepper

① In a large pan fry the onion and garlic in the oil for 5 minutes until softened but not browned. Add the grated carrot and chopped celery, then cover the pan and sweat the vegetables for 5 minutes.

② Add the butternut and the sliced carrots, and stir well. Add the stock and bring to the boil. Reduce the heat and simmer until the squash and carrots are tender, about 20 minutes.

③ Soya milk can be added near the end of cooking to make the soup a bit creamier, if you like. Season and liquidise until smooth.

Baked Fish with Rosemary Roasted Veggies

Fish is most nutritious when it is of the oily variety such as salmon, sardines or mackerel. Tuna is best avoided on a detox, however, due to its potentially high mercury content. For those who don't like the fuller flavour of oily fish, white fish can be substituted.

SERVES I

1 tsp olive oil, plus extra for brushing
1/2 red pepper, roughly chopped
1/2 celery stick, roughly chopped
1 courgette, roughly chopped
3 small tomatoes
3 shallots, quartered
1 garlic clove, finely chopped
sprig of rosemary
2 slices of lemon
175–225g (6–8oz) fillet of oily fish, such as salmon
freshly ground black pepper

① Preheat the oven to 180°C/350°F/Gas 4. Cut a piece of baking parchment large enough to hold the vegetables, and brush the inside with olive oil. Place the chopped vegetables and garlic onto the baking parchment. Drizzle over the 1 tsp olive oil and add a sprig of fresh rosemary. Fold over the edges to make a parcel. Place in the oven and bake for 10 minutes.

② Put 2 slices of lemon over the fish. Cut another piece of baking parchment large enough to hold the fish and brush the inside with olive oil. Wrap the fish in the baking parchment.

③ Put the wrapped fish onto a baking tray and bake for 10–15 minutes, or until the fish flakes easily with the tip of a knife. Remove the parcels, open onto a plate and serve.

Day 4

Greek Salad

Here is a traditional Greek, rough country salad of juicy tomatoes, crisp cucumber, sliced red onion, green pepper, crumbly feta cheese and plump olives. Serve this delightful combination with one of your lunch options, such as oatcakes or rice cakes.

SERVES I

3 tomatoes, cut into wedges or thinly sliced, or 6 baby plum tomatoes
1/4 red onion, sliced
1/2 cucumber, halved and thickly sliced
1/2 green or red pepper, thinly sliced
120g (4oz) feta cheese, cubed
8 olives

FOR THE DRESSING

1 tbsp extra virgin olive oil
1 tbsp linseed (flax) oil
1 1/2 tbsp lemon juice
1 garlic clove, crushed
1/2 tsp dried oregano
1/4 tsp freshly ground black pepper, plus extra to garnish

① To make the dressing, mix the olive oil, linseed oil, lemon juice, garlic, oregano and seasoning in a small jar with a screw-top lid and shake to combine.

② Place the salad ingredients in a large bowl. Pour the dressing over the salad and toss gently to combine just before serving. Garnish with a little freshly ground black pepper.

Variation

You can use a hard sheep's cheese such as Manchego instead of feta cheese, if you like.

Spanish-style Chickpeas with Wilted Spinach

Chickpeas are an excellent source of protein and are rich in calcium and iron as well as being a good source of fibre. They are versatile and have a delicious nutty flavour, which is really brought out in this tasty recipe. The recipe makes enough for you to use some for lunch on Day 5 as well.

SERVES 2
200g (7oz) dried chickpeas, soaked overnight, drained and rinsed, or 400g (14oz) can organic chickpeas, drained and rinsed
1 tbsp olive oil
1/2 onion
1/4 tsp ground ginger
1/4 tsp ground coriander
1/4 tsp freshly grated nutmeg
1 red pepper, chopped
1 red or green chilli, deseeded and finely chopped
225g (8oz) fresh tomatoes, chopped, or 400g (14oz) can chopped tomatoes
freshly ground black pepper
large handful of fresh spinach
chopped fresh coriander, to garnish

① Place the soaked and rinsed dried chickpeas, if using, in a pan, cover with water and bring to the boil for 15 minutes. Simmer for 1–1½ hours, or until the chickpeas are very tender. Drain and set aside.
② Heat the oil in a large pan and add the onion, spices, pepper, chilli and tomatoes. Cook over a low heat until the vegetables are tender, about 10 minutes.
③ Add the cooked or canned chickpeas and stir well. Add freshly ground black pepper to taste and heat through thoroughly, for about 5 minutes. Stir in the spinach and cook until it wilts. Garnish with fresh coriander and serve.

Day 5

Quinoa and Roast Vegetable Medley

Nutty-flavoured quinoa is a complete protein and goes very well with roasted onions, pepper, courgette and parsnip. There is enough of this delicious medley to serve for your lunch on Day 6.

SERVES 2

1 tsp olive oil, plus extra for brushing
3 shallots, or 1 sweet red onion, quartered
1 red or yellow pepper, chopped
1 courgette, chopped
1 small parsnip, or other seasonal root vegetable, chopped
55g (2oz) broccoli spears
1 garlic clove, crushed
1 tbsp fresh thyme
100g (3½oz) quinoa
250ml (9fl oz) vegetable stock (low-sodium variety or home-made)
1 tbsp chopped fresh parsley
linseed (flax) oil, for drizzling
freshly ground black pepper

① Preheat the oven to 180°C/350°F/Gas 4. Cut a piece of baking parchment large enough to hold the vegetables, and brush the inside with olive oil. Place all the chopped vegetables and the garlic onto the baking parchment and drizzle over the olive oil. Add the thyme leaves, season with black pepper and fold over the edges of the paper to make a parcel. Place the parcel in the oven and bake for 20 minutes.

② Put the quinoa in a pan and add the vegetable stock. Bring to the boil then simmer, stirring frequently, for about 10 minutes.

③ Cover the pan and take off the heat, leaving it to stand for a further 10 minutes.

④ Stir the roasted vegetables into the quinoa and add the parsley. Drizzle over some linseed oil and season with black pepper before serving.

Banana Ice Cream

This has got to be the simplest and healthiest banana ice cream ever – and it only takes moments to make once the banana has frozen.

SERVES 1
1 banana
75ml (2¹/₂fl oz) almond milk, or any other non-dairy milk
3 drops of vanilla extract
1 tsp maple syrup
carob powder or cinnamon, for dusting (optional)

① Peel the banana, halve it, then put it into a clear plastic freezer bag. Seal and place in the freezer until frozen. Take out the frozen halves and set them aside for a few minutes until they become slightly softer.
② Put the banana pieces into a food processor or blender and add the almond milk, the vanilla extract and maple syrup. Blend until smooth. Put into a serving bowl and decorate with a dusting of carob powder or cinnamon, if you like.

Day 6

Spicy Scrambled Eggs with Herb Salsa

A fresh herb salsa is a wonderful way to top piquant scrambled eggs. This is a nutritious dish as well as being full of flavour.

SERVES 1
2 organic eggs
3 tbsp soya milk
2 large tomatoes, chopped
¹/₂ tsp chilli flakes
2 tbsp fresh chopped coriander
freshly ground black pepper
1 tbsp olive oil
rye toast or oatcakes
wedge of lime, to serve

FOR THE HERB SALSA
1/2 400g (14oz) can diced tomatoes
1/2 green pepper, diced
1 onion, diced
handful of fresh coriander, chopped
1/2 tbsp chilli sauce
1 tbsp cider vinegar

① To make the herb salsa, in a bowl toss together the tomatoes, pepper, onion, coriander, chilli sauce and cider vinegar. Refrigerate for at least 30 minutes. Leftovers can be used for dips.

② Whisk the eggs, soya milk, tomatoes, chilli flakes, coriander and pepper together in a pan. Scramble this mixture with a little olive oil over a gentle heat for 3–4 minutes, stirring constantly with a wooden spoon.

③ Divide the egg mixture over rye toast or oatcakes and spoon over the salsa. Add a squeeze of fresh lime and serve immediately.

Day 7
Moroccan Avocado Salad

Crisp celery and salad leaves taste great with the warm flavour of walnuts and the sweetness of fruit. With the addition of avocado, this salad is full of healthy fats and cleansing, fresh ingredients.

SERVES 1
70g (2½oz) raisins or sultanas, or 5 fresh grapes, halved
½ celery stick, chopped
25g (1oz) walnuts, chopped
3 large handfuls of seasonal salad leaves
½ avocado, peeled, pitted and diced
½ apple, cored and chopped, or ½ orange, peeled and chopped
Life Detox Salad Dressing (page 135), to serve (optional)

① In a large bowl toss together the raisins or sultanas, celery, walnuts and salad leaves.

② Fold in the avocado and fresh fruit. Top with Life Detox Salad Dressing(page 127), if you like.

Sweet Potato Green Curry with Fish or Tofu

Fragrant Thai flavourings of lemon grass and kaffir lime leaves give a green curry its distinctive taste. It goes very well with sweet potatoes, green vegetables and fish – a healthy and delicious end to your detox week.

SERVES 1
1 small sweet potato or ½ large sweet potato
1 tbsp olive oil
½ tbsp green curry paste (see Cook's Tip below)
100g (3½oz) firm white fish or tofu, cut into chunks
handful of mangetouts, or other seasonal vegetable
1 kaffir lime leaf
1 lemon grass stalk
1 red chilli, deseeded and finely chopped
4 tbsp coconut milk
splash of yeast-free tamari

① Heat the oven to 180°C/350°F/Gas 4. Pierce the potato several times with a fork and place in the oven. Bake for approx 20–25 minutes, or until the flesh is beginning to soften. Set aside.
② Heat the oil in a pan and add the curry paste, stirring continuously. Add the fish or tofu, mangetouts or other vegetable, kaffir lime leaf, lemon grass and chilli. Cook over a low heat for 3 minutes.
③ Stir in the coconut milk and sweet potato, and simmer until the fish is cooked or the tofu is firm, about 7 minutes. Add a splash of tamari and serve.

Cook's Tip
Home-made green curry paste tastes much better than bought, if you have time to prepare it. The recipe on page 141 serves 4 people and will keep in the refrigerator for three days.

Green Curry Paste

MAKES ENOUGH FOR 4 PEOPLE
1 lemon grass stalk
2 tbsp ground coriander
1–3 green chillies, deseeded (depending on desired spiciness)
1 small onion, finely chopped
2 garlic cloves, crushed
1 thumb-size piece of fresh root ginger, peeled and sliced
2 kaffir lime leaves, cut into strips
1 bunch of fresh coriander, including stems
1½ tsp yeast-free tamari
a little coconut milk (if necessary)

Remove the tough outer leaves of the lemon grass stalk and cut off the bulb at the lower end. Use only the soft middle part and slice it finely. Place all the paste ingredients in a food processor or blender and blend until smooth. (If too dry, add a little coconut milk – just enough to keep the blades going.)

Banana Berry Bake

You can use any type of berry or a mixture to make this tasty bake. All berries are extremely good for you and frozen ones can be used when fresh are not available.

SERVES 1
handful of berries (frozen or fresh)
½ banana, chopped
1 tbsp flaked almonds
1 tsp desiccated coconut
natural yogurt or soya yogurt, to serve

① Preheat the oven to 180°C/350°F/Gas 4. Place all the ingredients in a small ovenproof dish and bake for 10–15 minutes, or until piping hot.
② Serve with a dollop of natural yogurt or soya yogurt. Dust with desiccated coconut if you like, and serve immediately.

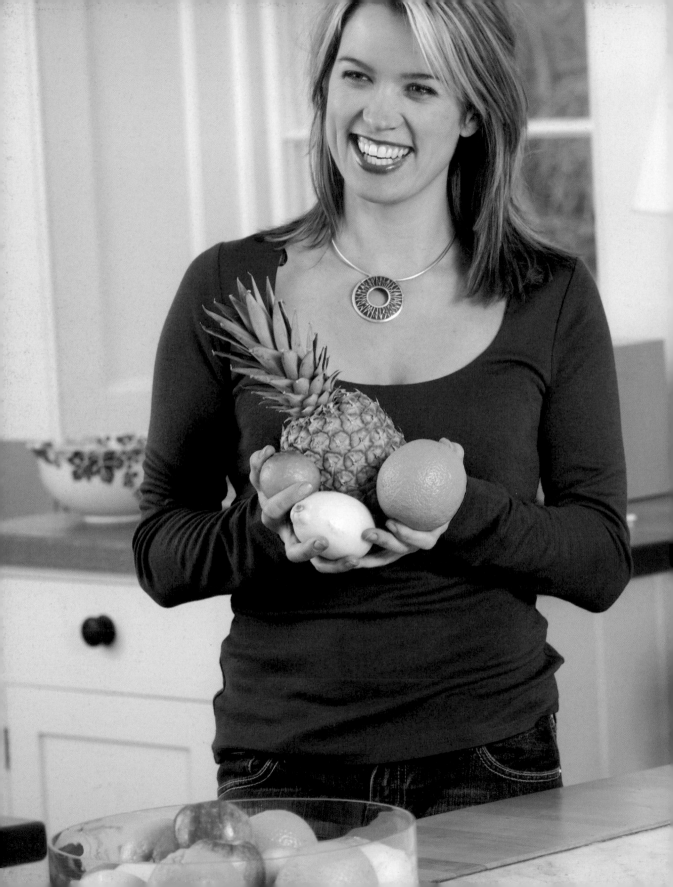

partthree®

living with
supreme
health and
happiness

chapter twelve

Immediately After Your Detox

Many people choose to add a turbo-detox day onto their 7-day programme. Not only are you in the detox frame of mind but also your body is primed and ready to push for optimum results.

'I lost 3 pounds in one day and feel fantastic – and I never even felt hungry!' Bryce, 36

The turbo-detox day is based on juice fasting. Fasting is an excellent way to remove unwanted toxins and weight very quickly and has been around for centuries. It is based on the principle that digestion takes up the vast majority of a body's energy, so, when this energy is freed up, it is used to heal, rejuvenate and rebalance the body. It is what your body naturally does when you are fighting off an illness: by reducing your appetite it obtains more energy for dealing with the illness.

Why juice fasting works best

Fresh juices provide the energy needed for optimum detoxification. Rather than starving the body, a juice fast feeds the system with high levels of vitamins and minerals. During a juice fast, the body has a chance to eliminate even greater amounts of toxins, so this is the perfect time for supportive therapies such as colon hydrotherapy.

The turbo-detox day is recommended *only* after the initial Life Detox 7-Day Programme is complete, in order that the body is well enough prepared. It is the ultimate pick-me-up!

Your 24-hour turbo-detox day

We do not recommend that you work during a 24-hour turbo-detox day – take the time out to help your body rest and for your mind to gain as much as possible from the process. Use the timetable below as a guideline only. As long as you consume the correct amount of juice and Life Detox Broth, you will be able take things at a pace that suits you. Choose a body booster, mind booster and mind detoxer exercise to do on your turbo-detox day from the 7-day programme. (Note: this 24-hour turbo detox is not recommended for any longer than the 24-hour period, because longer-term juice-fasting requires management from professionals – see retreats on page 154.)

Make the most of your turbo-detox day by following the steps below:

① We recommend that Juice Meals be consumed with 1 tsp of psyllium husks (see page 88).

② Juice Meals require 175ml (6fl oz) of liquid (or one small glass) and can be chosen from any of the juices from the 7-day programme.

③ Consume no less than 4 litres (7 pints) of water and 2 mugs of Life Detox Broth in the course of the 24 hours. Enjoy as much herbal tea as you like.

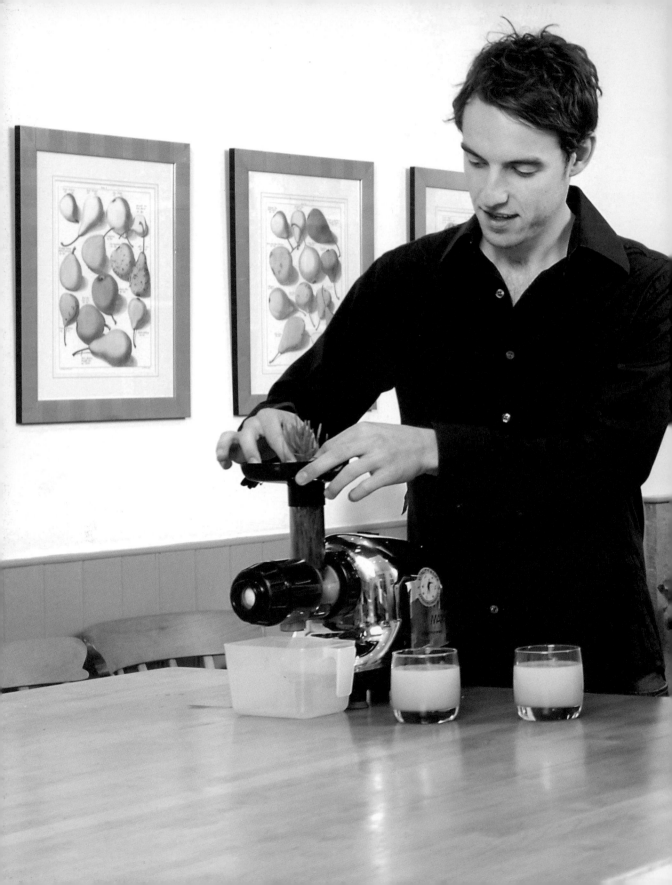

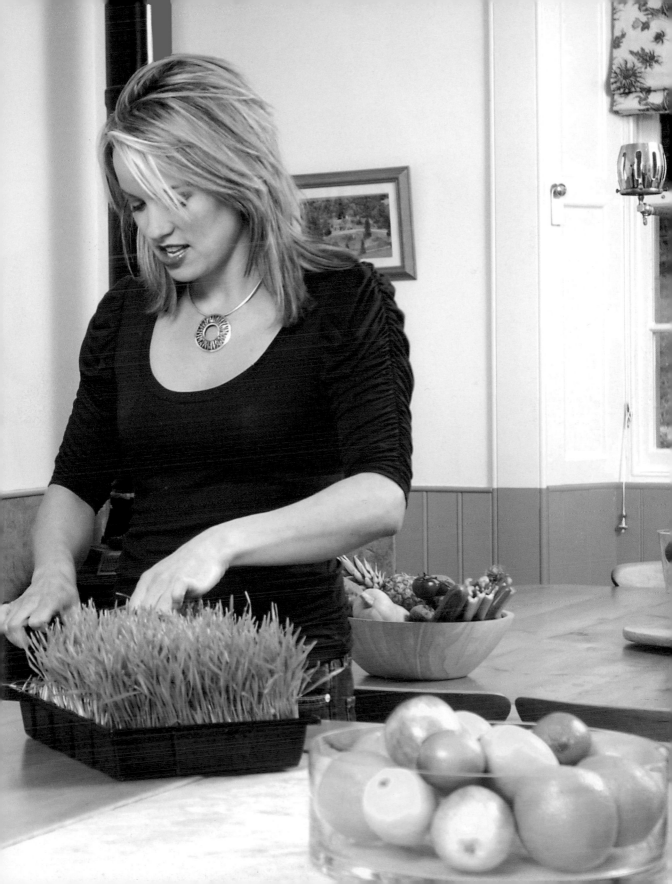

24-hour turbo-detox day schedule

8.15 am Power-up Process (page 82) followed by a cleansing drink of hot water with 2 slices of lemon

08.30 am 15-minute body exercise or booster of your choice

09.30 am First Juice Meal

10.00–11.00 am Mug of herbal tea

11.00 am–12.00 pm Choose which mind booster you would like to do

12.00 pm Second Juice Meal

12.00–6.00 pm A chance to go for a supportive therapy of your choice

1.30 pm Mug of Life Detox Broth (page 127)

3.00 pm Third Juice Meal

6.00 pm Fourth Juice Meal

7.00 pm Mug of Life Detox Broth (page 127)

8.00 pm Fifth Juice Meal

8.30 pm Do a mind detoxer exercise and booster of your choice

9.00 pm Herbal tea and Epsom salts bath (page 95)

Sustaining a Healthy Body and Mind

Sustaining a healthy body

We believe in enjoying life and I bet you do too. Being healthy in the long term plays a huge part in helping you enjoy all that life has to offer. However, we don't recommend becoming obsessive about food. If you are out for a fancy dinner where a delicious dessert is on the menu then enjoy it (without feeling guilty) and keep to our healthy guidelines the rest of the time.

It's all about balance

Your body works properly when you help it to maintain the best internal acid–alkaline balance. All food and drink is either alkaline-forming or acid-forming. By consuming the largest percentage of your diet from alkaline-forming or neutral foods and balancing the remainder with acid-forming foods, you can boost every aspect of your health and help to prevent problems.

It is based on a simple 80:20 rule:

The majority – 80 per cent – of your diet should be made up of alkaline-forming or neutral foods, and the remaining 20 per cent of your diet can consist of acid-forming foods. This is a vast improvement on most Western diets, which contain approximately 70 per cent acid foods. No wonder detox is needed. It is worth noting that some of the food in the acid-forming category, such as organic meat, fish or eggs, does still have health benefits. Nevertheless, it should not make up more than 20 per cent of your diet. If you are a big meat-eater, consider getting beneficial proteins from vegetable sources, found in the alkaline-forming food group.

Tips for making it easy

☺ Aim for one fifth of any meal plate to be made up of acid foods and the rest from the alkaline/neutral foods.

☺ Divide your daily meals into five servings, making just one of them from the acid-forming group.

It goes without saying that after doing a detox, you should stick to foods that pose less of a toxic threat, i.e. if eating meat or drinking milk, go for organic. Also, make sure you are not allergic or intolerant to the foods you are eating (see Suppliers and Further Resources for details of home testing kits).

See the dietary guidelines below for each of the categories and enjoy as much variety as possible within each food group.

80%: alkaline-forming/neutral foods

☺ All fruits and vegetables (including juices)

☺ Nut butters, nuts and seeds

☺ Pulses, beans and foods such as hummus (based on chickpeas)

☺ Grains such as rye bread, oatcakes, wholemeal bread, rice cakes and other wheat-free breads

☺ Essential fats (omegas 3 and 6; approx 2–3 tablespoons daily)

20%: acid-forming foods

Healthy options:

☺ Organic meat/unfarmed or organic fish

☺ Organic dairy products

☺ Organic eggs

Not healthy, treat with caution!

☹ Processed foods (including refined bread)

☹ Caffeine

☹ Alcohol

☹ Salt

☹ Carbonated drinks

☹ Sugar (either added to food or in processed foods)

Sustaining a happy mind

When was the last time you stopped to think about how amazing you are? Doing so is not only a nice feel-good thing to do, but it can have a massive impact on the quality of your life. People with a positive self-image tend to get more positive life results. It is therefore vital to nurture your relationship with yourself by remembering to give yourself a well-deserved pat on the back.

See the miracle in the mirror

So much has gone into making you and so much continues to happen to keep you being you. Just look at the following miraculous things about you:

☺ Your brain is more complex than the most powerful computer and has over 100 billion nerve cells.
☺ Your eyes can distinguish up to one million colours and take in more information than the largest telescope known to man.
☺ Your hearing is so sensitive it can distinguish between hundreds of thousands of different sounds.
☺ Your nose is the equivalent of a personal air-conditioning system, as it warms cold air, cools hot air and filters impurities.

Embrace the amazing new you. Every day you give birth to 100 billion new red cells and every year around 98 per cent of the atoms in your body are replaced. Today is a new day and you are an amazing new you!

Avoid living on autopilot

Slipping into autopilot as you go from one day to the next can severely limit your life enjoyment. If you don't notice all that you are and all that you have, it's hard to appreciate it and then you can't enjoy it properly. Take in the abundance, beauty and fun that exists in every moment. Become aware of everything you can see, hear, feel, smell and taste, right now. When you fully tune into the moment, you realise that nothing in the past is worthwhile thinking about and nothing in the future could possibly be any better than what you are being, doing and having, right now.

Adopt an attitude of altitude

Live your life without worrying about those things that so many people get stressed about: gossip, differences of opinion, deadlines, money, and so on. These things may continue to happen, but you can choose not to let them bother you.

Instead of reacting to situations based upon how you have reacted in the past, you respond to life events in ways that cause you the greatest amount of well-being and happiness.

You are more open-minded, present in each moment and purposeful in your actions. You no longer engage yourself with the daily dramas that so many people thrive on. Instead, you enjoy life from a higher perspective, where you see the bigger picture. With more understanding and compassion towards yourself and others, you live with an attitude of altitude.

Mind the gap

Setting goals creates a gap between where you are now and where you expect to be in the future. But you need to be careful to notice that the gap is there. Otherwise, it is easy to become focused on how things are not how you want them to be, and you end up feeling dissatisfied with your current set of circumstances. What often happens then is that you find yourself being very future-focused, and saying, 'I'll be happy when ...', which postpones your enjoyment of the magnificent moment.

When making changes to your body or life, instead of resisting your current set of circumstances, be mindful of, and accept, the gap. This way you focus less on improving and achieving all the time, and more on appreciating each moment, being kind to yourself and others and creating the best life possible. You know what you want, take actions consistent with your dreams and aspirations, and remember to enjoy the scenery along the way.

Feel your feelings

Check out the findings of the following incredible studies showing the health benefits of feeling your feelings.

In 1989, a study was published in the medical journal the *Lancet* showing a link between expressing emotions and the life expectancy of women with breast cancer.[11] The study involved 86 women who were undergoing treatment. Fifty of the women were randomly selected to have their care supplemented with a weekly support group. One of the main aims of the support group was to help the women express negative emotions such as sadness, fear and grief. Incredibly, on average, the women who attended the support group lived twice as long as the rest of the women involved in the study – an average of almost 18 months longer.

Also in 1989, James Gross of the University of California at Berkeley published findings which indicated that the speed of the progression of cancer tended to be faster in the patients who suppressed negative emotions.[11]

Although there are many different causes of cancer, and by no means are we suggesting negative emotions *cause* cancer, these studies nevertheless highlight that holding on to high levels of toxic emotions appears to be one factor that can speed up the progression of the disease. Instead of resisting your feelings, let yourself feel them and let them go.

Appreciate that less is more

People are beginning to realise that working hard to be, do or have more things often involves more stress. This is due to the time and effort required to manage, co-ordinate and protect more things. Illness and premature ageing can both be traced back to the wear and tear caused by excess stress and your body lacking time to relax and rejuvenate.

Do you need to simplify your life? In order for you to do this, you may need to give yourself permission to say no, if you genuinely don't want to do something. Acting out of obligation creates inner conflict that corrodes your peace and suppresses your joy. Instead, put yourself first. Think about this: if you are not healthy or happy, then how are you going to help someone else to be healthy or happy? It is possible to become so focused on trying to help others that you forget to help yourself. Putting yourself first is not selfish. It's about making choices and taking action based upon love and respect, rather than obligation.

You can enjoy life more by noticing more of the life you already have. We believe it is possible to reduce the number of needs you have to a point where you are fully nourished without needing a constant input of things to make you feel fulfilled. You will experience, perhaps for the first time, how effortless it is to sustain a happy mind when you notice, appreciate and enjoy your body and life for the incredible gifts they are, right now.

Treat yourself to an annual retreat

We hope you have enjoyed taking your Life Detox journey with us and will continue to enjoy the benefits of eating in a way that keeps your body in balance, as well as freeing your mind from toxic thoughts. If you want to take your detox further, one of our events might be ideal for you.

We run intensive detox events around the world. These specialist events last between three and ten days and take place at stunning retreat locations. If you are in need of rejuvenation of your mind, body and spirit then this could be your next step.

On our Life Detox retreat, people regularly lose 7–14lb (3.2–6.4kg) in one week – this dramatic weight loss is a combination of fat loss and the removal of impacted waste matter from the colon. These retreats have a more intensive detox programme and require our specialist management. Juice fasting and colon cleansing are two of the mainstays of the managed detox, coupled with yoga, a full range of wonderfully relaxing complementary therapies and experts on hand to guide you and take care of your every need. Our events are fun, informative and give you the tools and knowledge you need to help integrate detox into your life. Visit www.lifedetox.co.uk and click on 'retreats' if you would like to treat your body and mind.

Notes

Chapter 1

1. Ian Sample, 'Chemical World', *Guardian*, 22 May 2004, p. 4.
2. 'Vinyl Products Expose Children to Toxic Additives', *Greenpeace*, 15 June 2001
3. Blandford, T.B., Seamon, P.J., Hughes, R., Pattison, M. and Wilderspin, M.P., 'A case of polytetrafluoroethylene poisoning in cockatiels accompanied by polymer fume fever in the owner', *Veterinary Record*, Vol. 96 (8), pp. 175–8.
4. telecomworldwire, 5 May 2000
5. American Society for Reproductive Medicine, 21–25 October 2006, Poster 398

Chapter 2

6. Will Knight, NewScientist.com, news service, 13:42, 5 January 2004
7. NIH Publication no. 06–949 February 2006, National Institute of Diabetes & Digestive & Kidney Diseases, US Department of Health and Human services
8. www.foresight-preconception.org

Chapter 3

9. Rein, G., Atkinson, M. and McCraty, R., 'The physiological and psychological effects of compassion and anger', *Journal of Advancement in Medicine*, Vol. 8 (2), 1995, pp. 87–105
10. McCarthy, R., Atkinson, M., Tiller, W.A., Rein, G. and Watkins, A.D., 'The effects of emotions on short-term power spectrum analysis of heart rate variability', *American Journal of Cardiology*, Vol. 16 (14), 1995, pp. 1089–93

Chapter 13

11. Spiegel, D., Bloom, J.R., Kraemer, H.C. and Gottheil, E., 'Effect of psychosocial treatment on survival of patients with metastatic breast cancer', *Lancet*, 14 October 1989, pp. 888-891
12. Gross, J., 'Emotional expression in cancer onset and progression', *Social Science and Medicine*, Vol. 28 (12), 1989, pp. 1239–48

Picture Credits

p. 12: Gul Kaynak.
p. 15, pp. 56–7, p. 66, p. 89, p. 142, pp. 146–7: Malcolm Cochrane.
Illustration pp 28–9: Simon Pearsall.
p. 33: Gary John Norman/Getty Images.
p. 44: Michelangelo Gratton/Getty Images.
pp. 72–3, p. 108: Sandy Newbigging and Amanda Hamilton.
p. 81: Anthony Johnson/Getty Images.
p. 84: Stuart McClymont/Getty Images.
p. 95: Siri Stafford/Getty Images.
p. 101: Maria Teijeiro/Getty Images.
p. 110: Louis Fox/Getty Images.
p. 113: Matthew Wakem/Getty Images.
p. 119: Leigh Beisch/Getty Images.
p.120: Jonelle Weaver/Getty Images.
p. 129: Lisa Romerein/Getty Images.

Suppliers and Further Resources

**UK and International Detox Retreats
by Life Detox:**
www.lifedetox.co.uk, Tel.: 0845 500 7545
Food Intolerance Testing Kits by Yorktest:
York Laboratories, York Science Park,
York, YO10 5DQ, UK
www.yorktest.com, Tel.: 0800 074 6185
**7-Day Home Detox Kit, detox support
formula (specialist liver supplement,
colon support supplements, skin brushes
and enema kits from:**
Nutrigold
P.O. Box 13289, Birmingham, B30 9BB, UK
www.nutri-gold.com, Tel.: 0845 603 5675
Email: talk2us@nutrigold.co.uk
**Fresh wheatgrass, barley grass, psyllium
husks and other health-related products
(including rebounder trampolines) from:**
Juiceland
Unit 86, Hartlebury Trading Estate,
Hartlebury, DY10 4JB, UK
www.juiceland.co.uk, Tel.: 01299 250009
Email: enquiries@juiceland.co.uk
Many of these items can also be bought
at health-food shops.
Juicers (including masticating) from:
Get Juicing
6 Reynolds Drive, Oakengates, Telford,
TF2 6NG, UK
www.getjuicing.com, Tel.: 01952 277324
A wide range of juicers is also available
from good kitchenware shops and
department stores.
Natural skin care and cosmetics from:
Living Nature UK
Unit 6, Gardeners Business Park, Sherfield
English Lane, Plaitford, Hants, SO51 6EJ, UK
www.livingnature.com, Tel.: 01794 323222

Barefoot Botanicals Limited,
201 Dyke Road, Brighton, BN3 1TL, UK
www.barefoot-botanicals.com
Tel.: 0870 220 2273, Outside UK tel.:
+44 1273 823031
**Home-made natural skin care
by Pamplemousse:**
Contact: Hala Sioufi
Email: pamplemousse_douce@hotmail.com
Infrared Sauna by Physiotherm, from:
MagMed Ltd, 3 Willetts Court, Pottergate,
Norwich, NR2 1DG, UK
www.physiotherm.net, Tel.: 0845 225 5008
In Australia:
Physiotherm Australia, MagMed Ltd, Suite 1,
10–12 Blackburn Road, Blackburn, VIC 3130,
Australia. Free-phone. 1 800 060 088
In New Zealand:
Physiotherm NZ, MagMed Ltd, 153
Lochhead Rd, RD6, Tauranga, New Zealand
Free-phone 0800 624 633
Non-toxic household cleaning products:
Mypure
www.mypure.co.uk, Tel.:0845 456 0639
Ecover (available worldwide)
www.ecover.com
**Alternatives to garden pesticides,
see Pesticide Action Network UK:**
www.pan-uk.org
**Colonic Hydrotherapy, see The Association
and Register of Colon Hydrotherapists:**
www.colonic-association.org
Tel.: 0870 241 6567
**Complementary therapists in your
area, see Complementary Therapists
Association:**
www.complementary.assoc.org.uk
Tel.: 0870 201 1912

Index

Amanda Hamilton

For information about the work Amanda and Sandy do together, please visit www.lifedetox.co.uk

Amanda has been a successful nutritionist for many years, running clinics throughout Europe. She founded a specialist retreat company called 'Life Detox Retreats' to help people rejuvenate their body and mind – with the help of some of the world's leading therapists – at stunning locations around the world. Visit www.lifedetox.co.uk for information on how you can attend a life-changing retreat. Amanda is also in high demand as a TV presenter and public speaker. Visit www.amandahamilton.co.uk for more information.

Sandy Newbigging

Sandy combines ancient principles and practices with cutting-edge therapies and techniques to help people from around the world to enjoy the body and life they want. You can meet with Sandy for a one-to-one consultation at either of his clinics in Edinburgh or London, at one of his retreats throughout Europe or by attending one of his popular workshops. His other books include, 'New Beginnings' and 'Wisdom without Waffle'. Visit www.sandynewbigging.com for more information.